Clinical Skills in Neurology

Michael J.G. Harrison DM FRCP

Professor in Clinical Neurology,
University College London Medical School
Consultant Neurologist,
Middlesex Hospital and National Hospital,
Queen Square, London

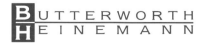

Butterworth-Heinemann
Linacre House, Jordan Hill, Oxford OX2 8DP
A division of Reed Educational and Professional Publishing Ltd

ℛ A member of the Reed Elsevier plc group

OXFORD BOSTON JOHANNESBURG
MELBOURNE NEW DELHI SINGAPORE

First published 1996
Reprinted 1997

British Library Cataloguing in Publication Data
A catalogue record for this book is available from the British Library

Library of Congress Cataloguing in Publication Data
A catalogue record for this book is available from the Library of Congress

ISBN 0 7506 2520 1

Typeset by Keyword Typesetting Services Limited
and printed and bound in Great Britain by Cambus Litho Ltd, East Kilbride

Clinical Skills in Neurology

Contents

Introduction

This book sets out to show the clinical student at whatever stage of their career how to take and interpret a neurological history and especially how to examine the nervous system. It attempts to provide a practical approach to the common neurological problems and describes the basic investigations used in making a diagnosis. I hope it goes some way to demystifying the whole subject.

Much of the text is freely borrowed from the earlier *Neurological Skills* but much is new. I again would like to acknowledge the insights gained from my clinical teachers, colleagues, junior staff, students and patients. Many ideas are public property, appearing in other texts many of which are acknowledged in the brief reference lists.

To simplify the text, the patient has been referred to as 'he' throughout, although cases occur in both sexes. In order that subsections can be consulted in isolation, there is some repetition of key points.

Acknowledgements

It is a pleasure to record my gratitude to Sheila Sellars and Geoffrey Smaldon of Butterworth-Heinemann and to Teresa Fullam, who patiently oversaw the revisions of the manuscript. Professor L Luxon, Dr A Lees, Dr Clare Fowler, Dr Steve White and Mr J Brazier kindly read parts of the text and made many helpful suggestions. Dr Margaret Hall Craggs and Dr Brian Kendall kindly provided some of the illustrations in the account of cerebral and spinal imaging.

1

History and examination

The history

Taking a revealing history is a highly skilled exercise. Although it is learnt largely by apprenticeship, some advice can be proffered, and practice with audio-visual recording can be helpful in the early stages.

It is important to secure the patient's trust from the outset and to allay his nervousness by a friendly approach and due privacy. A history taken in the open ward is unlikely to be given in a relaxed way, and so may be unreliable. The examiner must hide his irritation at vagueness and his hurry. The patient must feel that *this* doctor will listen, and has time to hear him out. It is vital to look and appear interested. Greet the outpatient at the door, shake his hand, introduce yourself, and invite him to join you seated at your desk. Sit him at the side, not across the desk in the job interview position. If students are sitting in on the consultation be sure their presence is acceptable to the patient. If you are that student explain that the senior doctor who will be seeing him has asked you to do the 'preliminary detective work', if he is agreeable. It may then be helpful to indicate the purpose of the consultation if it is the result of a referral letter — 'your doctor has asked me to have a think about these unpleasant dizzy turns you have been having'.

Establish eye contact, and by your body language indicate that you are sensitive to the distress of whatever symptoms may be set before you. Do not remain totally silent. 'Mms' and head nodding encourage the patient to relax and tell his story. If he starts to ramble, however, it is equally important to bring him gently back onto the subject. All this means that a mental note must be made of matters that will eventually need clarification by gentle probing. Initially the patient must be allowed to get off his chest those things he most wants the doctor to hear about. Later, it is also appropriate to discourage a catalogue of second-hand medical opinions from previous consultations, and to analyse what the patient has meant by words like numb, or dizzy. However, care must be taken not to 'lead the witness' by suggesting answers to important questions. It can be helpful to ask 'anything else?', and 'how are things at home?', to trigger discussion of matters that the patient was perhaps semi-reluctant to proffer by himself. To gauge the severity and impact of problems one should ask if the symptoms interfere with normal activities, including work, hobbies and sleep. Ask what the patient can no longer do since the advent of the presenting complaint. By showing interest and sympathy at this stage one is also building a rapport that will not only be vital to the patient's compliance with advice or medication, but also to his trust in the diagnosis.

As one listens it is important to start theorising about the meaning of the history taken. What is the anatomical implication of the presenting symptom or group of symptoms; does it sound like a disorder of consciousness, of the vestibular or visual systems, of motor or sensory function, etc.? The hypothesis should only be vague but it will be important in directing the later questions aimed at clarification, and at confirming or refuting the initial localization. For example, if it sounds as though the patient may have spinal cord disease, one would go on to ask about back pain and sphincter disturbance if these had not yet been mentioned.

As well as giving clues about the function or part of the neuraxis at fault, the history also reveals most of the information needed to diagnose the nature of the pathological process responsible for the symptoms. Thus the nature of the onset and the time course of evolution of symptoms reveal whether the patient has a vascular or mechanical lesion (sudden onset), an inflammatory disease (usually subacute onset over days) or a neoplastic or degenerative disorder (insidious onset with progressive deterioration). Intermittent processes like those in multiple sclerosis, epilepsy and migraine produce a diagnostically episodic history (see Figure 1.1).

The history also directs the subsequent examination. At the end of the history it should be clear which parts of the neurological examination are going to be crucial. The examination 'digs' where the history has marked an 'X', or rather a '?'. In addition the examiner will be intent on ruling out other possibilities, as well as confirming the first hypothesis. Alternative diagnoses that require very differ-

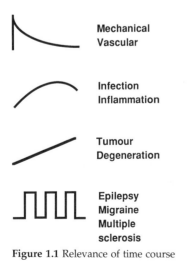

Figure 1.1 Relevance of time course

Mechanical
Vascular

Infection
Inflammation

Tumour
Degeneration

Epilepsy
Migraine
Multiple
sclerosis

ent management or treatment must always be considered, if only to be refuted. It is helpful to ask yourself the question whether the evidence points to a focal problem (stroke, tumour, multiple sclerosis), or to a diffuse problem (toxic, metabolic, degenerative).

Certain symptoms point to particular problems. Thus if a patient complaining of muscular weakness describes difficulty getting out of a car, getting off the toilet, rising from a deep chair, getting up from a kneeling position, lifting their children or working above head height, a proximal distribution of affected muscles is likely, and the patient may well have muscle disease. If, by contrast the patient describes tripping, dragging of their feet, wearing out of the toes of their shoes, a poor grip, and dropping things, a distal weakness is being described and the patient is more likely to have a peripheral neuropathy. Weakness confined to the legs immediately suggests spinal disease. An additional report of a band, girdle, belt, or tightness around the chest or abdomen suggests a sensory level due to cord disease. Cranial nerve dysfunction is suggested by complaints of diplopia, facial numbness or weakness, deafness or dizziness, or dysarthria and dysphagia. Cerebellar localization is indicated by complaints of staggering, walking in a drunken fashion, having difficulty with putting a key into a lock, lighting a cigarette, and writing. Radiculopathy is suggested by pain down the limb, with exacerbation on head turning or leg stretching.

It should be clear that history taking is an active process, the examiner processing the information, formulating a hypothesis or several hypotheses, rejecting some as further data appear, and planning the examination. Research has shown that the experienced clinician makes his first hypothesis, albeit a fairly vague one, within seconds of meeting the patient.

The clues are not only those of the stated history. Whilst the patient is being greeted, seated, and invited to explain his problem, the clinician has an opportunity to start the examination. The patient reveals much of his personality, mood, intelligence, memory, language, and voice as he tells his story. Body language is also revealing. The patient's agitated or depressed mood affects his movements. His dishevelled state may indicate dementia or alcoholism.

Some neurological conditions may be suspected on first meeting the patient. The walk as the new patient approaches the desk may reveal parkinsonism, hemiplegia, ataxia, or foot drop. The difficulty getting out of the chair at the end of the interview may alert one to the possibility of proximal muscle weakness. The general appearance of the face may suggest an endocrine abnormality (hypopituitarism, acromegaly, hypothyroidism, exophthalmic goitre) or reveal a rash (adenoma sebaceum, lupus pernio, disseminated lupus erythematosis, dermatomyositis). Erosion of the nasal bridge may indicate Wegener's granulomatosis. All such observations are clues to the neurological condition. A parkinsonian immobility or a weak face may be obvious and disorders of the eyelids or eyes can be noticeable as the patient is questioned. A tilt of the head may suggest cervical disc disease, a posterior fossa tumour, or diplopia due to weakness of one of the oblique muscles. Parkinsonian tremor may become obvious in the hand resting on the lap. Tics, restless movements of the legs (akathisia), and other involuntary movements may be noticeable.

Note taking should be limited and saved until later, usually to the interval when the patient is getting undressed. If the doctor has his head in the case folder and is scribbling furiously, his patient is unlikely to relax and fully co-operate, and some valuable physical signs may be missed. Some shorthand notes may be necessary in a complex story if the chronology is important.

The act of making a diagnosis is frequently one of pattern recognition. The patient who describes sharp stabs of pain in one side of the face provoked by eating and talking, who gives the history without moving his mouth more than a fraction, and who points to the site of the pain without daring to touch the pointing finger on the face, has trigeminal neuralgia. Such a spot diagnosis is not often possible, however, and routine questions are needed both of nervous system function, and of the health of other systems (Table 1.1).

Some routine questions will also reveal important occupational risks (toxic neuro-

Table 1.1 Routine neurological enquiry

Have you noticed any change in your mood, memory or concentration?

Is your sleep disturbed?

Have you had any black-outs or been dizzy? Have there been any problems with vision, hearing or balance?

Have you had difficulty with talking, chewing or swallowing?

Have you noticed any numbness or pins and needles in your face, body, arms or legs?

Have you had weakness, heaviness or clumsiness of your limbs?

Is your walking affected?

Have you normal control over your bowels and waterworks and is sexual function normal?

pathy), travel exposures (parasitic infections), abuse of alcohol, tobacco and recreational drugs, genetic factors (muscular dystrophies, cerebellar degeneration, Huntington's chorea), and relevant past illnesses and treatment (head injury, meningitis, steroids, etc.), all of which may be crucial to a neurological diagnosis. Some information about home circumstances and the patient's support network may prove valuable when considering how he will cope with a serious diagnosis or taxing treatment.

Problems in the interview may arise because the patient is unintelligent, dementing, has hearing loss, is depressed or frightened, or has a language disorder (dysphasia). The doctor may be tired, have a headache, be inattentive or interrupt too often. If not careful he may put words into his patient's mouth in an attempt to save time and cut corners. The solution may be to start again on another occasion. All junior doctors know the irritation of hearing a patient produce a new gem of information when telling his story to the consultant, which he forgot or was insufficiently encouraged to reveal when first encountered. The other aid to overcoming these difficulties is to interview a relative as well. Besides confirming the accuracy of the patient's own story, such additional history may also reveal the patient's lack of memory or a change of personality. Eyewitness accounts of attacks of loss of consciousness, for example, are worth miles of EEG recording, so patients with black-outs must be asked to bring an eye-witness to the consultation if at all possible. A phone call to a relative, workmate or doctor may not be a glamorous way of making a diagnosis but can be very 'cost effective'.

Some features of the history suggest that the patient will be unlikely to have any evidence of organic disease. The patient may show either exaggerated distress, or demonstrate 'la belle indifference'. A shopping list of medical consultations or symptoms, or a bizarre symptom, may arouse suspicions in the clinician's mind. Discrepancies may also be obvious in the patient's appearance. A woman with difficulty in using her hands is unlikely to be accurately made up. Well brushed hair may conflict with a complaint that the arms cannot be lifted above shoulder level.

Finally, one should recall probabilities. Most headaches will be due to migraine or tension, for example. This does not mean that other important causes must not be considered and excluded but it does mean that the clinician's 'bias' should be towards the likely, not the unlikely. The other guiding principle is to not miss a treatable disease. To this end subdural haematoma, thyroid and B_{12} deficiency, and hypoglycaemia all warrant consideration above their statistical rating.

When the examination is over and a plan of action is being formulated, it is crucial to explain to the patient what you believe the matter to be, what tests are going to be necessary, and whether they are confirmatory or, in less clear-cut circumstances, exploratory. The need for some tests to rule out serious diseases even when they are not very likely should also be explained. When at this or a subsequent visit a diagnosis is named it is vital to discover what the patient understands by concepts like a stroke (often held to be a kind of heart attack). What the disease is not due to (stress, work, etc.) may be more important information for the patient than a detailed account of recent research into molecular biology to explain the condition. Remember to tell patients when they do not have brain tumours, multiple sclerosis, Parkinson's disease and stroke. They may have harboured such fears ever since they were told they were being sent to a neurologist. Always

attempt to give a prognosis, though it is reasonable to explain that the art of prognosis is often more difficult than that of diagnosis. If treatment is prescribed, try to indicate how it is going to work, what can be expected of it, and what it is not going to do. Mention important side effects and whether they are to be worked through, reported, or require immediate cessation of treatment. Finally say what your role, if any, is going to be in the following months or years. At the very end ask if the patient or any accompanying relative has any other questions. Stress that you will give their usual medical attendant all necessary details, and wish them well.

Further reading

BALLA, J.I. (1980) *Pathways in Neurological Diagnosis*. Edward Arnold, London.

The general examination

The routine physical examination including obligatory measurement of the blood pressure may of course reveal the cause of neurological problems but will not be considered in detail. Clearly a hard prostate, a breast lump, lymphadenopathy, a cardiac source of embolism or signs of organ failure may all be crucial. Some aspects of the examination are more directly relevant to the making of a neurological diagnosis, however, and will be discussed.

Some diagnoses are immediately suggested — so-called 'spot' diagnoses. The stork-like legs of Charcot–Marie–Tooth disease, the neurofibromata of von Recklinghausen's disease, the head of Paget's disease, the puckered mouth of scleroderma, the rash of lupus, and the eye signs of thyroid disease are examples. More often, the findings have to be elicited by careful scrutiny. The skull should be palpated for lumps or bulges (over a meningioma), its circumference measured if hydrocephalus is suspected, and it should be percussed. A cracked-pot note suggests open sutures, for example in an infant with hydrocephalus, and unilateral dullness may indicate a subdural collection. In an older person the superficial temporal arteries may be reddened, thick, tortuous, and non-pulsatile due to giant cell arteritis.

The spine too is percussed for focal tenderness suggesting local pathology such as an epidural abscess, or vertebral metastases, and observed and palpated for any hint of scoliotic curvature. Such a curve may be congenital or part of a hereditary condition such as Friedreich's ataxia, but may also be acquired from muscle paralysis as in poliomyelitis or with skeletal disease. A tuft of hair or dimple in the lumbar region may be a clue to a congenital spinal abnormality such as spina bifida.

The size of the two hands and feet should be compared by placing them side by side. A hemiparesis in infancy may be reflected in retarded growth on one side. The length and girth of thumbs or fingers, or the length and width of the foot may reveal a difference. The patient may know that he needs a half size smaller shoe on one side. A high arched foot under which a light can be seen from the side even when a flat board is pressed up onto the heel and sole can be a sign of other congenital anomalies or hereditary conditions. Such a pes cavus is found, for example, in some hereditary neuropathies. The toes tend to be bunched up.

Examination of the skin may yield useful clues. Many café-au-lait patches (more than five) and axillary freckles are indicative of neurofibromatosis even when there are no obvious fibromas or neuromas. Inherited on chromosome 17, type 1 has the risk of optic nerve glioma, mental retardation and seizures. The rarer type 2 causes bilateral acoustic neuromas. A rash on the face may indicate tuberose sclerosis, in which subependymal hamartomas may develop into astrocytomas, and the patient may have seizures, mental retardation, subungual fibromas, retinal, renal, and cardiac tumours. A facial rash is also seen in dermatomyositis with muscle pain, tenderness, and weakness. The fine pale texture of the skin of a patient with pituitary failure may prompt a survey of body hair and testicular size. A port-wine stain on the forehead due to a naevus may be associated with an intracranial cortical vascular malformation which may cause epilepsy and a hemiparesis (Sturge–Weber syndrome). Telangiectasia, for example in the conjunctivae, may be associated with ataxia, involuntary movements, and a history of infections with very low levels of IgA (ataxia telangiectasia). Nail folds or the tips of digits may reveal small infarcts due to vasculitis, pertinent in the investigation of neuropathies, for example. Nail clubbing in the absence of congenital heart disease makes carcinoma of the lung a possible cause for a cerebellar syndrome, cerebral metastases, or paraneoplastic neuropathy. Organomegaly in the abdomen raises suspicions of carcinomatosis, lymphoma, or haematological or even storage disease, all of which may yield a neurological diagnosis.

Thyroid gland enlargement may be the clue to hypothyroidism or thyrotoxicosis as the cause of myopathies, neuropathies, eye signs, or tremor, etc.

Neck stiffness is sought by passive flexion of the neck by the examiner's hands under the occiput. This is best done from directly in front of the patient with the examiner's elbows flexed. Limitation suggests meningitis or subarachnoid bleeding. If lateral flexion of the neck is restricted, cervical spondylosis is the likely cause. A general rigidity is felt in some parkinsonian syndromes. Limitation of elevation of the extended leg with the examiner's hand under the heel implies root irritation, for example by a prolapsed disc, or meningeal irritation. If the flexed knee is brought up to the abdomen and the knee is then extended, resistance is felt again with meningism or root entrapment (Kernig's sign). Tight hamstring muscles may limit straight leg raising but any pain is restricted to that muscle.

A bruit may be heard over cranial arteriovenous malformations or fistulae; it is best sought by placing the bell of an 'old-fashioned' stethoscope over the closed eye. The patient should be asked to open the other eye and fix his gaze so that movement of the eyeball under the stethoscope does not cause uninvited extraneous noises. Bruits over the neck commonly arise from the heart. If this is the case they will be recognized over the precordium and heard in the sternal notch and will fade out somewhat as they are conducted up the major vessels. A bruit restricted to the angle of the jaw is likely to be a marker of atheromatous stenotic disease of the carotid artery. Venous hums have a lower frequency, vary with head position and posture, and may be stopped either by gentle pressure on the neck or a Valsalva manoeuvre. A thyrotoxic goitre may also be the source of a continuous murmur. Auscultation over the spine may extremely rarely reveal the bruit of a spinal angioma, and is worth carrying out in patients with a spinal lesion.

Joint disease may impair movement and complicate testing of muscle power so the full range of passive movement at joints like the shoulder and knee may have to be checked. Swelling and abnormal mobility may be found in a Charcot joint, disorganized by loss of pain sensibility as in syringomyelia, tabes dorsalis or diabetes mellitus.

The neurological examination

Mental state and language

The patient's appearance, demeanour and performance during history-taking are themselves good tests of intelligence, memory and behaviour. Whilst the history is being given it may become clear that the patient is anxious, depressed, thought disordered, confused, amnesic or overtly demented. More formal assessment may need the skills of a clinical psychologist but an intermediate level of testing at the bedside by the clinician is an important part of the neurological examination.

Dysphasia

Listening to the patient's speech and observing his comprehension of what he hears will give an impression of language capability. This is preferable to trying to take a short cut and testing naming ability, which can be mildly defective in confused patients when it does not prove that the dominant hemisphere is damaged. The ability to read, write and repeat words and phrases should be tested. Lesions in the frontal lobe produce a non-fluent disturbance of speech. The patient comprehends normally but produces few words or telegrammatic short sentences. Phrases are usually less than four words. The speech lacks melody and rhythm, and is effortful. Prepositional speech is lost before expletives. Little grammatical words like 'to' and 'from' are lost. Singing, counting, and reciting letters of the alphabet may be relatively spared. Because Broca's area for speech is close to the face and mouth area of the motor strip, there may be some difficulty pronouncing some syllables due to a 'high level' disturbance of complex muscle activity needed for articulation. Smaller frontal lesions may produce a similar disturbance but with preserved ability to repeat phrases given to the patient (transcortical motor aphasia).

When there is a temporal lobe lesion causing dysphasia the speech is fluent though full of errors and low on informational content (Wernicke's aphasia). Many words are incorrect (paralogisms) and some are apparently newly invented ones (neologisms). The normal cadence of speech is preserved (prosody) and the patient sounds as though he is talking in an unfamiliar language. To add to this impression he fails to understand the spoken word. Parieto-occipital lesions may produce a similar disturbance but with preserved repetition (transcortical sensory aphasia). Extensive lesions of the dominant hemisphere may affect both the temporal and frontal areas involved in language function. The resultant global dysphasia is non-fluent and the patient is also unable to understand. Rare disconnections of these two speech areas, for example by lesions in the parietal lobe, produce a fluent dysphasia with relatively preserved comprehension but a great difficulty in repeating phrases (conduction aphasia) (Table 1.2).

Table 1.2 Types of dysphasia

Type	Site	Output	Comprehension	Other
Broca	Frontal	Non-fluent	Good	Hemiplegia
Transcortical motor	"	"	"	Can repeat
Wernicke	Temporal	Fluent	Bad	Field loss
Transcortical sensory	Parieto-occipital	"	"	Can repeat
Conduction	Parietal	Fluent	Good	Can't repeat

Mutism

Total mutism may accompany the onset of Broca or global aphasia, but may also be seen after head injury, immediately after a seizure, or be due to a reaction to phenothiazine.

Other faculties

The detection of any type of dysphasia defines a lesion in the dominant hemisphere which, in some 95% of the population, is on the left. Other neuropsychological deficits that implicate the left hemisphere include difficulties with calculation and verbal memory. Right-sided lesions should be suspected if the patient has lost visual memory, has difficulty with visuospatial tasks such as dressing and finding his way, or shows striking neglect or denial of the left side (anosognosia).

Frontal lobe lesions cause personality change with apathy or disinhibited silliness. The patient may be incontinent and may have a grasp reflex — when the examiner draws his fingertips down the palm and on to the palmar aspect of the patient's fingers they curl to grip his hand against an adducted straight thumb. A subfrontal tumour such as a meningioma may cause telltale anosmia, or optic atrophy on one side (the side of the mass) and papilloedema on the other — the Foster–Kennedy syndrome. Seizures are common in frontal lobe disease and often versive in type with head and eyes usually turning away from the side of the irritative lesion. Status epilepticus in a patient who has never had a fit before is often due to a frontal lobe lesion.

Temporal lobe lesions are characterized by memory problems, Wernicke aphasia, visual field defects and seizures affecting smell, taste, visual, auditory or bodily sensations. Parietal lobe lesions cause difficulties with performance of complex acts (praxis) such as striking a match, despite adequate muscular power and co-ordination. On the non-dominant side a special difficulty with dressing may occur and denial and neglect of the opposite limbs are likely. Recognition of faces may be impaired. On the dominant side, difficulty with calculations, right-left orientation and writing are seen (Gerstmann's syndrome). A lesion of the left angular gyrus causes striking difficulty with reading. Contralateral sensory disturbance is usually detectable.

Occipital lobe lesions, as well as causing field defects, impair colour recognition and the identification of objects from their visual image (visual agnosia). Bilateral damage to the visual cortex causes blindness with loss of optokinetic nystagmus. The patient may deny blindness (Anton's syndrome).

Table 1.3 sets out the neuropsychological 'scan' which provides localising evidence. Global impairment of such functions, especially of learning and memory, imply dementia. Simple tests of general knowledge, the ability to calculate, learn a name and address and recall it after 3 minutes, as well as the learning and reproduction of an abstract Binet figure will reveal modest impairment. Severe degrees of dementia are obvious when the patient cannot name the day and date, identify where they are, or give an account of themselves. Formal psychometry is necessary when there is any uncertainty, especially when there is a problem in distinguishing depression from dementia. A mini-mental state examination can be used to quantitate moderate dementia at the bedside (Table 1.4).

Table 1.3 Neuropsychological deficits

	Left hemisphere	Right hemisphere	Either/both
Frontal	Verbal fluency (Broca aphasia)	'Silent'	Either: Incontinent, adversive seizures, grasp reflex, difficulty shifting strategy (perseveration) and in problem solving, disinhibited or flat/apathetic Both: Demented
Temporal	Verbal memory Verbal comprehension (Wernicke's aphasia)	Visual memory recognizing faces	Either: Visual field defect, facial weakness, *TLE (smells, taste, visual or auditory hallucinations, epigastric sensation, fear, lip-smacking, grimace) Both: Severe amnesia
Parietal	Dyscalculia right-left confusion dysgraphia conduction aphasia	Neglect/denial dressing dyspraxia getting lost	Either: Constructional apraxia, sensory deficit, inattention, demented
Parieto-occipital	Dyslexia	Agnosia for faces	Either: Colour vision impaired, visual agnosia, field defect
Occipital			Either: Field defect Both: Occipital blindness ± denial (Anton's syndrome)

*TLE = Temporal Lobe Epilepsy.

Table 1.4 The mini-mental state examination

Orientation – 1 point for each correct answer
  What is the:
    time
    date
    day
    month
    year   5 points (   )
  What is the name of this:
    ward
    hospital
    district
    town
    country   5 points (   )
Registration
  Name three objects
  Score 1,2,3 points according to how many are repeated
  Re-submit list until patient word perfect in order to
  use this for a later test of recall.
  Score only first attempt   3 points (   )
Attention and calculation
  Have the patient subtract 7 from 100 and then from the
  result a total of five times. Score 1 point for each
  correct subtraction   5 points (   )

Recall
  Ask for the three objects used in the registration test, one
  point being awarded for each correct answer
                                              3 points (   )
Language
  One point each for two objects correctly named (pencil
  and watch)   2 points (   )
  One point for correct repetition of 'No ifs, ands and buts'
                                              1 point (   )
  3 points if three-stage commands correctly obeyed 'Take
  this piece of paper in your right hand, fold it in half,
  and place it on the floor'   3 points (   )
  1 point for correct response to a written command such
  as 'close your eyes'   1 point (   )
  Have the patient write a sentence. Award 1 point if the
  sentence is meaningful, has a verb and a subject
                                              1 point (   )
  Test the patient's ability to copy a complex diagram of
  two-intersected pentagons   1 point (   )

Total score 30

N.B. This score is a useful bedside assessment of dementia. It should not be used to test for focal psychological deficit, being heavily weighted on verbal performance. See discussion in Journal of Neurology, Neurosurgery and Psychiatry 1984, B47, 496–499.

Confusion superficially resembles dementia but the history is short and the patient is agitated and hallucinated. His attention span is short, and conscious level mildly impaired. There is rich detail in confused answers, unlike the paucity of the replies of the demented. There is usually an obvious underlying cause, e.g. pneumonia.

Further reading

GOODGLASS, H. (1993) *Understanding Aphasia*. Academic Press, San Diego.
DEVINSKI. O. (1992) *Behavioural Neurology: 100 Maxims*. Edward Arnold, London.
WALSH, K.W. (1991) *Neuropsychology. A Clinical Approach*, 2nd edition. Churchill Livingston, Edinburgh.

Cranial nerves

The thoroughness with which cranial nerve function needs to be assessed depends a great deal on circumstances. If symptoms are confined to cranial nerve territories then each will need detailed testing.

On the other hand, if a hemisphere lesion is suspected one should concentrate on the visual fields, the optic fundi, horizontal eye movements, facial sensation and movement, and head turning to either side. The sense of smell is only really of importance after head injury and, for example, in the case of a possible frontal tumour, suggested by personality change, dementia, or adversive fits. The corneal reflex needs to be tested if the 5th nerve is symptomatic, if a cerebellopontine angle tumour is suspected or if other cranial nerves are faulty. The testing of taste is rarely crucial and testing the gag reflex only relevant when there are bulbar symptoms or other lower cranial nerve functions are affected.

1st — Olfactory nerve

Subtle testing requires the use of different 'smells'. The neurological tray often contains numerous bottles carrying exotic labels — cloves, roses, peppermint, etc. After a brief stay in the ward cupboard they are usually indistinguishable. Asafoetida retains its pungent nastiness and the patient's recoil is proof that he has not had his olfactory bulb sheared away in a head injury. It is more practical to see if the patient can smell coffee or an orange from a patient's locker. One nostril is occluded with a finger and the item brought towards the patient, who has his eyes closed. As soon as he registers the smell he then attempts to identify it. Before testing smell it is necessary to check that the airway is clear by first asking the patient to sniff through either nostril. A complaint of distorted smell without loss may be a depressive symptom. Loss, if not due to nasal disease, is usually due to trauma, rarely to a frontal meningioma or other tumour. Meningitis or subarachnoid haemorrhage are seldom the cause. Heavy smoking dulls the sense of smell and patients with Parkinson's disease, multiple sclerosis or Alzheimer's have also been shown to have impairments.

2nd — Optic nerve

Examination of the fundus

The visibility of the retina and optic disc provides a unique opportunity for direct inspection of arterioles and venules, and of a central nervous pathway.

Skill in visualizing the optic disc and retinal vessels and in interpreting pathological changes comes from practice. Clinical students are advised to examine the fundi of all patients, however unlikely it is that their observations will be relevant to the presenting complaint, if only to train their own eye by building up a personal bank of data on the normal appearances. If necessary, the fundi can be observed through the patient's own spectacles to aid focusing when there is a large refractive error. The optic disc can be located by following a vessel as it gets larger until the disc edge is reached. Fixation on a distant object by the patient holds the fundal structures still while they are observed. This requires co-operation by the patient, and the observer cannot expect a successful fixation if he puts his head in the way of the view of the other side of the ward or the ceiling. The right eye must be examined with the right eye from the right side of the bed or couch, and the observer must learn to use his left eye to examine the patient's left eye from the left side of the couch to avoid covering the line of sight of the unobserved eye. The examiner should try to keep his 'unused' eye open which helps to prevent accommodation of his viewing eye. The room should be dim, so that the pupil is large. Mydriatics should not be used routinely. The upper lid may have to be held up by the examiner to clear his view, but remember to tell the patient you are going to do it!

The normal fundus [Plate 1.1 (a,b)]

The normal optic disc, lying to the nasal side of the posterior pole of the eye, is circular and

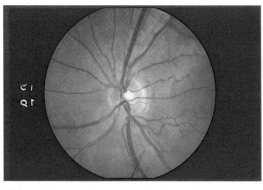

(a)

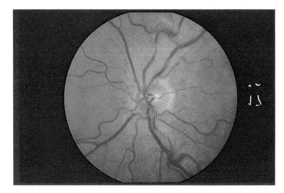

(b)

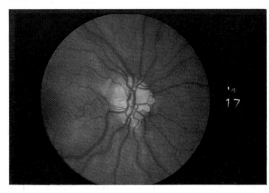

(c)

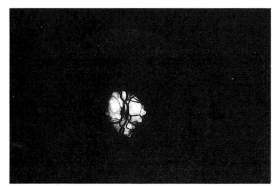
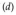

(d)

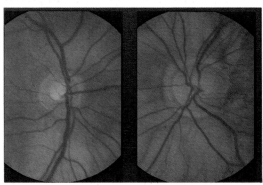

(e)

Plate 1.1 *(a)* and *(b)* Normal left fundus. Note the normal cup, the slight pinkness of the disc, and the clear margin and normal calibre of the arteries and veins. The veins appear darker and straighter than the smaller arteries. There are no exudates or haemorrhages. The macula region on the right of the picture is of a darker colour. *(c)* Drüsen of the right disc which may cause confusion due to resultant blurring of the disc margin often misinterpreted as papilloedema. Note their bunch-of-grapes apearance. *(d)* Autofluorescence of drüsen. No fluorescein has been injected, but the picture was taken with fluorescein filters in the camera. *(e)* Myopic fundus on the right contrasted with normal fundus on the left. The disc of the myopic is larger, a little paler, and surrounded by a rim of peripapillary atrophy. The rest of the fundal background also looks patchy owing to thinning of the choroid.

pale pink in colour, rather paler than the surrounding retina. The edge of the disc is clear, although not as well demarcated on the nasal side as on the temporal side. The nasal side looks rather pinker than the temporal side.

The physiological cup from which the vessels emerge is visible as a well-defined depression in the nerve head. It is of paler colour than the peripheral rim of the disc which has more vessels on its surface. It is usually no more than 40% of the whole disc and is symmetrical with the cup in the opposite disc. The rest of the fundus has an even red background due to the presence of blood in the choroid. If there is little retinal pigment, the variegated choroidal pattern shows through as a 'tigroid fundus'. In patients with myopia the choroid may be thin and the fundus looks pale with patches in which the white sclera is visible. When the retinal pigmentary layer has more pigment in it the fundus looks brown. Great variations in the colour are thus encountered, many being the results of racial differences.

Crossing the fundus from the disc are the retinal arteries and veins. The calibre of the arteries is usually two-thirds that of the veins. The blood in the arteries appears a brighter red than the more purplish hue in the veins. The arterial wall is not normally appreciated, the colour and form being that of the column of blood. The veins on the disc can often be seen to pulsate, but the lack of such pulsation is not necessarily pathological. From the temporal side of the disc small cilioretinal vessels may be seen running towards the area of the macula.

The macula lies some 1.5–2 disc diameters from the disc on its temporal side. It is free of major retinal arteries and veins and is of a darker red colour, because the choroid shows through more readily in the central area that is devoid of nerve fibres.

Small colloid bodies (drüsen) may be seen buried in the disc (Plate 1.1 (c) and (d)). They are of importance since they give the disc an appearance that may be mistaken for papilloedema. They can be recognised by their bunch-of-grapes appearance which is usually best detected at the disc edge, their autofluorescence, and the lack of signs of diffuse oedema after intravenous fluorescein. If they are buried papilloedema is closely mimicked and

only a fluorescein angiogram can make the distinction.

Hypermetropic individuals have smaller, pinker discs. Myopic subjects have larger paler discs, commonly with a white crescentic area to one side — the myopic crescent [Plate 1.1(e)].

Optic atrophy (Plate 1.2)

Damage to the optic nerve causes loss of myelin sheaths around individual fibres, variable degrees of secondary gliotic scarring, and loss of the capillary bed within the nerve head. These changes cause pallor of the optic disc on which the diagnosis of optic atrophy depends. The cause may be toxic, compressive, or demyelinating in type, all with the same effect on the appearance of the disc.

The disc looks paler than normal, standing out in greater contrast from the red background of the rest of the fundus. The lamina cribrosa is often more than usually clear and the limits of the physiological cup are easy to define. The edge of the disc itself looks sharp. When the atrophy is severe the disc is paper-white and may shrink to a shallow excavation with a punctate appearance due to the perforations of the lamina cribrosa.

Lesser degrees of atrophy can be difficult to detect. The disc is normally paler in infancy and old age. With most causes of atrophy the change is more obvious on the temporal side of the disc. The nasal side usually looks pinker because of the concentration of vessels there, so temporal pallor is an exaggeration of the normal appearance. It is difficult to be sure of the significance of such a change in any individual unless there is visual loss or a field defect to confirm the pathological nature of the changes seen. There may be less than the usual number of vessels visible on the edge of the disc. Experienced observers claim that less than seven confirms atrophy.

Visual loss parallels the loss of fibres and the pupil response to light may be impaired. Visual evoked responses may be delayed, diminished, or absent.

Secondary changes in the metabolic demands of the retina may lead to a non-specific narrowing of the arterial lumen in the

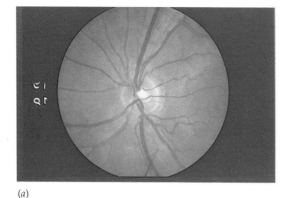

(a)

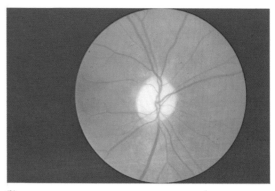

(b)

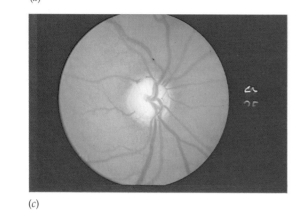

(c)

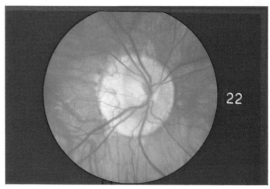

(d)

Plate 1.2 (a) Normal fundus. (b) Very pale disc in a case of optic atrophy. The whole right disc is pale and a cup is visible. The edge appears stencilled owing to enhanced colour contrast between the pale disc and the normal retina. There are no arterial changes to suggest a vascular aetiology in this particular case. (c) A deep cup due to glaucoma may make the disc look pale. Here the enlarged cup is detected by the peripheral position from which vessels emerge close to the rim of the right disc. (d) High myopia also makes the disc look paler than normal. Here the right disc looks larger than normal, and the patient has a refraction error.

presence of optic atrophy. Such vessel changes are obviously more prominent if the optic atrophy is the result of retinal infarction, for example due to central retinal artery occlusion (see p. 14).

Protracted papilloedema may lead to optic atrophy. In this situation the disc as well as looking paler than normal still has a blurred edge and a filled-in physiological cup. Later

on the blurring disappears, and the appearance is indistinguishable from primary optic atrophy.

Myopic subjects have a paler than normal disc and much experience is needed at times in distinguishing the presence of optic atrophy in a severely myopic individual.

The enlarged cup of glaucoma can give the disc a paler than normal appearance. The size of the cup may be seen from the position of the emerging retinal vessels and then the colour of the peripheral rim of the intact disc can be checked. Glaucoma may cause optic atrophy, therefore this distinction is an important one.

Papilloedema (Plate 1.3)

Oedema of the optic nerve head (optic disc oedema) occurs with local lesions such as optic neuritis or as a result of raised intracranial pressure (ICP) in which case it is correct to call it papilloedema. In this condition the

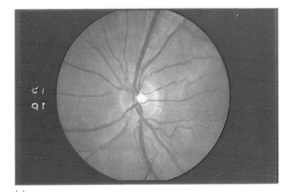

(a)

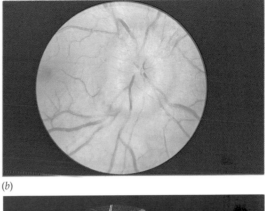

(b)

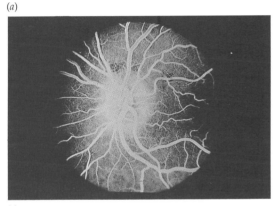

(c)

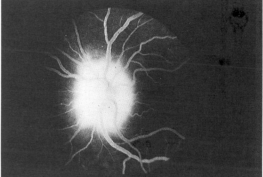

(d)

Plate 1.3 (a) Normal fundus. (b) Disc oedema due to raised intracranial pressure. The margin of the right disc is lost, vessels run forward to clear the elevated edge, and the disc surface is hyperaemic with more visible small vessels and a pinker than normal colour. There is no visible cup. There are no haemorrhages or exudates to suggest malignant hypertension. (c) Fluorescein lights up the left disc head 16 seconds after injection when the arteries and veins of the retina are filled. (d) At 5 minutes residual fluorescein that has left the vascular compartment owing to the local breakdown of permeability to serum albumin is seen in the disc head.

appearance of the disc shows several changes. It becomes pinker than usual and approximates more closely to the colour of the retina. The veins become enlarged, particularly with papilloedema of rapid onset, and lose their pulsation. Venous pulsation is commonly but not always seen in the sitting position and its loss is not necessarily patho-

logical. Its preservation is unusual with papilloedema and should make one question the diagnosis.

As the disc head becomes more oedematous the definition of the lamina cribrosa is lost and the physiological cup becomes filled in. Occasionally, the cup is retained and the swollen disc edge gives a conical look to the elevated disc. The edge of the disc becomes blurred, especially on the nasal side, which is normally less distinct in any case. The vessels leaving the disc appear elevated and when the oedema is severe they seem to emerge from a soft mass. An increased number of small vessels can be seen on the surface of the disc. Haemorrhages and exudates may appear on or near the disc edge. If the elevated ICP is chronic and unrelieved, secondary optic atrophy causes some pallor of the still-blurred disc and the retinal arteries become narrower. Until this happens visual acuity is unaffected except momentarily on changes of posture. Papilloedema does not affect the pupillary reflex.

Differential diagnosis

Optic neuritis is distinguished by early visual loss and central field defect. Pallor develops rapidly. Malignant hypertension causes disc oedema, but the associated haemorrhages are disproportionately florid and widespread and there are other arterial changes and exudates. The blood pressure is elevated.

Congenital anomalies of the disc may cause confusion but venous pulsation is usually present. Hyaline bodies or drüsen, if buried on the nerve head, make it appear swollen. Their presence can be suggested by their bunch-of-grapes appearance on the disc margin. Hypermetropic discs in long-sighted people look pinker than normal, making the differential diagnosis of early disc oedema more difficult in such subjects.

Fluorescein injected as an intravenous bolus can be followed through the retinal circulation with an ophthalmoscope or retinal camera using appropriate filters. The sequential arrival of dye in arteries, capillaries and veins can be appreciated. The retinal equivalent of the blood–brain barrier restricts the albumin-bound fluorescein to the vascular compartment in the normal eye. In the presence of papilloedema the barrier is broken down and fluorescein leaks into the disc; fluorescence of the disc head persists for many minutes after the injection.

Retinal artery occlusion [Plate 1.4(b–d)]

Central retinal artery occlusion causes a sudden loss of vision in one eye. The arteries appear collapsed and pale. The retina is pale and indistinct or cloudy due to oedema in the nerve-fibre layer. Only the macula retains its usual pink appearance because of the absence of nerve fibres in that area. By contrast with the milky colour of the fundus the macula looks redder than normal and is known as the cherry-red spot. After a few weeks the ischaemic oedema of the retina subsides and the cherry-red spot 'fades'. Stasis in the retinal arteries may be obvious with cattle-trucking or breaking up of the column of blood on the

venous side. Subsequently, the arteries become sheathed in appearance and attenuated. The optic disc becomes pale due to optic atrophy following death of ganglion cells in the infarcted retina. If the patient has a large cilioretinal artery, the macula and its neighbouring retina may be spared. There may be a retained island of central vision in such cases, and the normal colour of the cilioretinal vessel and its area of supply stand out in clear contrast to the rest of the fundus.

The occlusion of a retinal artery branch, usually due to embolism, causes an appropriate focal area of retinal infarction and oedema. An occluding embolus of a cholesterol crystal or calcific heart valve debris may be visible in the occluded vessel. Cholesterol emboli may also be seen in asymptomatic eyes because the birefringent crystals can impact in a vessel without obstructing all of its lumen. These yellow shiny bodies look larger than the vessel in which they are caught. They are due to the discharge of atheromatous debris from ulcerated plaques in the aorta or carotid artery.

Platelet fibrin emboli arising as mural thrombi on similar atheromatous lesions may be seen fleetingly as white bodies traversing the retina. They are commonly the cause of attacks of transient loss of vision in one eye (amaurosis fugax).

Retinal vein occlusions (Plate 1.5)

Occlusion of the central retinal vein is frequently associated with hypertension. In the severe case all the veins in the affected fundus are congested, dilated, tortuous and accompanied by haemorrhages. The haemorrhages are scattered throughout the fundus. They are dark and irregular but may lie alongside the congested veins. The haemorrhages may be so extensive as to make it impossible to see further details of the fundus. Some of the haemorrhages may break through into the vitreous. The arteries at first seem unaffected, although it may be difficult to see them. In milder cases with less florid haemorrhages, oedema of the retina and optic disc may be obvious. Patchy exudates are prominent due to areas of retinal ischaemia as a result of capillary closure. The veins are dilated, tortuous and darker than usual. Central retinal vein occlusion occurs at

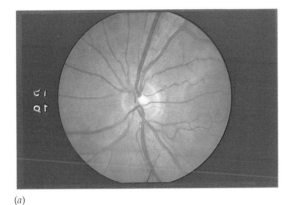

(a)

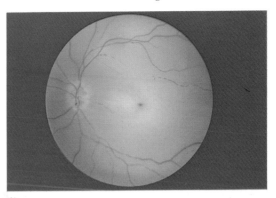

(b)

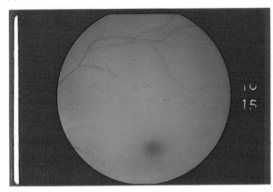

(c)

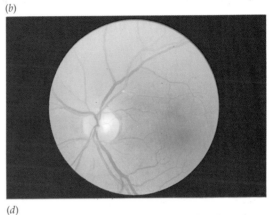

(d)

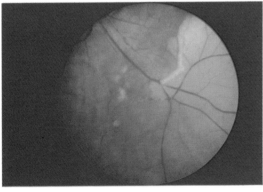

(e)

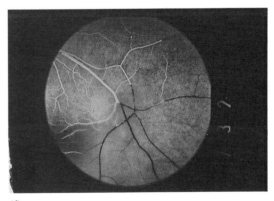

(f)

Plate 1.4 (a) Normal fundus. (b) Central retinal artery occlusion in the left eye. There is pallor of the retina except at the macula which therefore stands out as a cherry-red spot. The vessels are narrow. (c) Close-up of the occlusion in *Plate 1.4(b)*. There is segmentation of the column of blood (cattle-trucking) due to stasis. (d) Cholesterol embolus in the superior temporal branch of a retinal artery at a point of bifurcation in the left eye.

(e) Branch occlusion of a retinal artery. There is the same evidence of stasis in the artery. The upper right third of the visible retina is infarcted and pale. (f) Fluorescein shows patency of the vessel proximal to a point of obstruction. Venous filling occurs only on the left from intact retina. There is no capillary blush in the infarcted area.

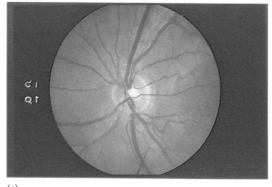

(a)

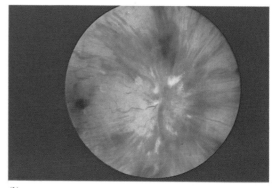

(b)

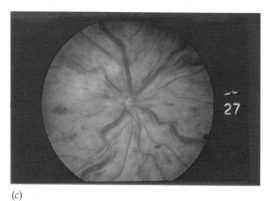

(c)

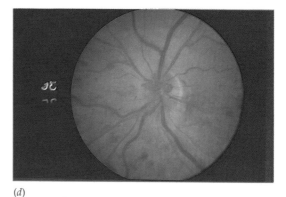

(d)

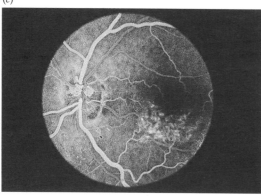

(e)

Plate 1.5 (a) Normal fundus. (b) and (c). Examples of right-sided central retinal vein occlusion showing dilated tortuous retinal veins, widely distributed retinal haemorrhages, and disc oedema. In some cases capillary closure is a prominent feature and cotton-wool spots predominate. (d) Hemispheric venous occlusion in the left eye. The changes of venous obstruction are confined to the lower half of the retina. Collateral channels are visible on the disc. (e) The fluorescein angiogram shows leakage in the venous phase.

the level of the lamina cribrosa and is often accompanied by sudden severe visual impairment. Secondary changes include arterial narrowing and sheathing, glaucoma in up to 20% of cases, and the development of new venous channels. Venous collaterals may be seen in tortuous coils overlying the disc.

Occlusion of a branch of a retinal vein produces venous congestion and haemorrhages confined to part of the retina. The site of occlusion often appears to be at a venous–arterial crossing. Vision is only likely to be seriously affected if the macula area is involved. In hyperviscosity syndromes bilateral changes can be seen with dilated veins but few haemorrhages and less retinal oedema. Vision is therefore usually spared.

Hypertensive retinopathy (Plate 1.6)

In 1939 Keith, Wagener and Barber proposed a classification of hypertensive retinal appearances which is still useful. In groups 1 and 2 fell patients with changes confined to arterioles. Group 3 consisted of those with haemorrhages and exudates. In group 4 they placed anyone with superadded optic disc oedema.

In younger patients diffuse narrowing of arterioles is commonly seen; in older people the narrowing is segmental. The earliest change in calibre is reversible, although it is due to arterial thickening with medial hypertrophy. Other segments are dilated with associated medial atrophy. The thickened walls give a heightened light reflex, appearing more like copper or silver wire. Veins may show nipping at points of arterial crossing. These early changes may be seen in normotensive individuals with arteriosclerosis. With increasing severity of hypertension retinal haemorrhages and exudates make their appearance. The haemorrhages lying in the nerve-fibre layer are flame shaped and often lie close to the disc.

Soft exudates appear initially as a greyish area but rapidly develop into a cotton-wool spot, frequently half as big as the disc itself. They may arise singly or in clusters, and often, although they surround the macula, it is spared. They are due to an area of capillary closure with retinal microinfarction. The cotton-wool spot fades and fragments over approximately 6 weeks. Fluorescein leaks from the area of a cotton-wool spot and demonstrates micro-aneurysms, often in the region of the areas of capillary closure.

Deeper, waxy hard-looking exudates are more common near the macula (macula star). These may persist.

In group 4 retinopathy the arterial changes, haemorrhages and exudates are accompanied by disc oedema. The disc is reddened, swollen and crossed by dilated capillaries which leak fluorescein. The differential diagnosis includes papilloedema, but in that condition haemorrhages and exudates are less florid and more restricted to the area immediately around the disc.

Diabetic retinopathy (Plate 1.7)

Mild background retinopathy consists initially of microaneurysms, dilated capillaries, small haemorrhages and areas of capillary closure with cotton-wool exudates. Fluorescein angiography often reveals many microaneurysms that are too small to be seen by the naked eye. In maculopathy, hard exudates, micro-aneurysms or haemorrhages affect the macular area which becomes oedematous and in turn affects visual acuity (6/12 or worse). The hard exudates appear to encircle the fovea centralis and move in on it. Fluorescein shows areas of missing capillary loops and microaneurysms that leak. Areas of non-perfusion appear to stimulate new vessel formation in the retina or in front of it, that is proliferative retinopathy. The new vessels resemble fans or fronds of a broad-leafed plant. They often develop on the optic disc but may appear anywhere in the periphery. When overlying the macula they cause severe visual impairment. Vitreous tends to adhere to the retina at points of new vessel formation; with shrinkage of the vitreous there is a risk of haemorrhage from the new vessels and areas of mechanical retinal damage. Connective tissue proliferation may follow new vessel formation, and advanced diabetic eye disease consists of vitreous haemorrhage, retinal detachment and fibrous change.

The scars of photocoagulation treatment for proliferative retinopathy have a characteristic moon-crater appearance.

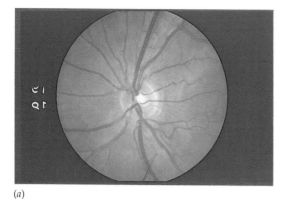

(a)

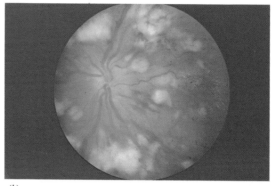

(b)

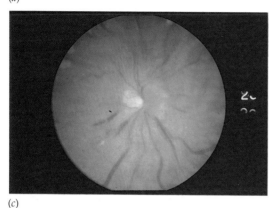

(c)

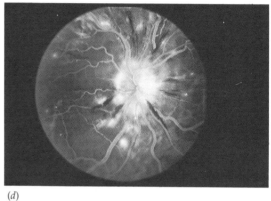

(d)

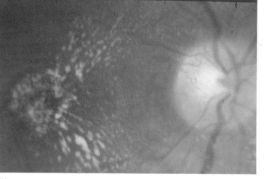

(e)

Plate 1.6 *(a)* Normal fundus. *(b)* Hypertensive retinopathy. The left fundus shows linear haemorrhages and cotton-wool spot exudates. There is also disc oedema. *(c)* Disc oedema in another case of malignant hypertension, here seen in the right fundus. Note the streaky haemorrhages and peripheral exudates. *(d)* The leak after fluorescein injection is not confined to the disc. The features of *Plates 1.6(c)* and *(d)* help to distinguish malignant hypertensive retinopathy from papilloedema due to raised intracranial pressure. *(e)* Hard exudates which in this case have formed a star at the right macula.

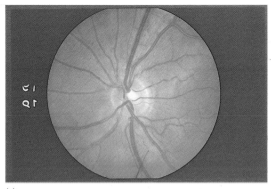
(a)

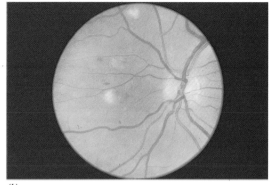
(b)

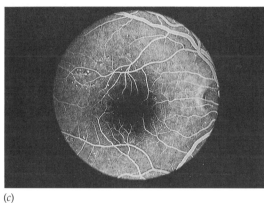
(c)

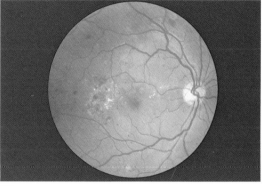
(d)

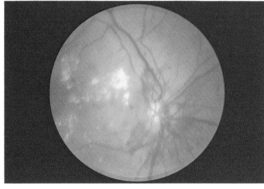
(e)

Plate 1.7 (a) Normal fundus. (b) Diabetic retinopathy. Microaneurysms, small blot haemorrhages, and yellowish exudates are also present in the right fundus. (c) Fluorescein angiogram of the same fundus. (d) There are more extensive waxy exudates in this right fundus. (e) Neovascularization in a diabetic with a typical frond-like arrangement of the new leash of vessels close to the left disc.

Visual acuity and visual fields

It is surprising how frequently visual acuity is forgotten and no record of it appears in the assessment of even those patients whose primary complaint is of loss of vision. The two standard techniques involve firstly the optician's chart where the patient should be allowed to guess at the line below the one at which they baulk. Each eye is tested in turn and the acuity is conventionally recorded as 6/6 or 6/9 when the chart is viewed from 6m. In the USA the distance is 20 feet and the vision recorded as 20/20, for example. The size of the letter on the chart denoted by '24' or '36' (acuity 6/24 or 6/36) is that which would at 24 or 36 m subtend the same angle as the smaller letters denoted by '6' do at 6 m.

The person with poor visual acuity of say 6/36 is thus seeing at 6m what they should be able to see at 36 m. If the patient is ill in bed a small chart can be hand held at 1.5 m (Figure 1.2)

This testing should be supplemented by reading test types e.g. those of Jaeger, when most people can read between J1 and J4. It is obviously important that any error of refraction is corrected before interpreting a difficulty as proof of an abnormality of the retina or optic nerve. Often patients have forgotten to bring their spectacles to the consultation, even when they know they are coming about their failing vision! Getting the patient to look through a pinhole, if necessary made on the spot in an appointment card, can be a useful way of correcting modest errors. The best acuity achieved is obviously the best guide to the neurologically relevant acuity. If acuity is too bad to read the largest of test type, i.e. worse than 6/60, the ability to count fingers, see hand movements, or perceive light should be recorded.

Visual field testing can be done to varying degrees of thoroughness. If a simple assessment is needed to exclude a hemianopia, e.g. in a patient with headache or epilepsy, but in whom there is no stronger reason to suspect a field defect, the following abbreviated techniques may suffice. The patient is confronted and the examiner holds both extended arms above the visual horizontal axis and asks the patient to look at the bridge of the examiner's nose. The index finger of each hand is moved quickly once and the patient asked to report movement on the left, on the right or on both sides. The test is repeated below the horizontal (Figure 1.3). If all four stimuli are picked up the patient is unlikely to have a hemianopia or quadrantanopia or the inattention in a half-field that may occur with parietal lobe lesions. This short-cut way of testing will miss nasal

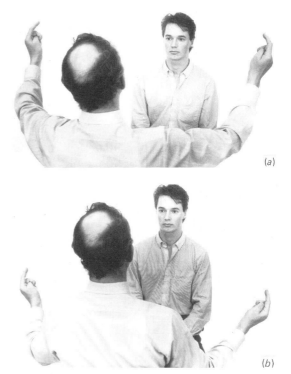

Figure 1.3 Visual field testing by confrontation. The patient looks directly at the examiner's nose and says where he sees a movement of either or both hands, both above (a) and below (b) the horizontal. This screening method only detects major field loss and misses rare nasal field defects and scotomas.

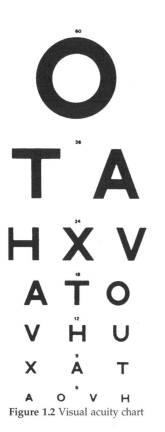

Figure 1.2 Visual acuity chart

field defects and will not be adequate if there are visual symptoms or a high index of suspicion of a defect. Then confrontation using a 5 mm white hat pin should be carried out sitting opposite the patient whose single uncovered eye has to keep its gaze on the examiner's eye. The pin is brought in at arm's length from most directions on the clock and the patient reports each time it appears. A red pin may be needed to detect a restriction in the smaller red field, e.g. in chiasmatic lesions. A small circumscribed defect in the central field, a 'scotoma', can be detected using a small 1 mm white or red pin. This can also be used to map the blind spot, the 'physiological' scotoma due to the lack of retinal elements at the site of the optic nerve head. The size of the blind spot reflects the size of the head of the optic nerve so it is enlarged in the presence of papilloedema.

In drowsy, confused and dysphasic patients when co-operation with confrontation is not possible, the blink response to a menace from either side is compared, to test for a hemianopia. A finger is advanced rapidly towards the undefended cornea from either half-field. The open hand should not be used as the draught it produces may provoke a corneal reflex which may be misconstrued as a response to an object in the visual field.

Retinal lesions cause lost acuity throughout the field of one or both eyes, or in a sector appropriate to a part of the retina affected, for example an altitudinal hemianopia if a branch of the central retinal artery is occluded. With retinal microvascular damage, for example in glaucoma with raised intraocular pressure, a bundle of retinal nerve fibres may be affected producing an arcuate scotoma. With field defects of retinal origin the causative lesion is visible on ophthalmoscopy which helps to distinguish the cause of something like an altitudinal hemianopia which can also arise by infarction of the optic nerve. As no vessel crosses the horizontal meridian retinal vascular defects always honour that boundary.

The commonest lesion of the optic nerve is an acute optic neuritis (retrobulbar neuritis), and the history is characteristic **(p. 84)**. The visual loss may affect the whole field or often the maximal loss is central with fibres

from the macula preferentially affected by demyelination in the optic nerve. A central scotoma results. Colour discrimination is lost and may never return though acuity usually recovers. Subtle asymmetries of pupil responsiveness may be detectable (see below). Compression of the optic nerve, though rare, must be detected early if sight is to be saved by timely neurosurgical intervention. The early fall in acuity may be accompanied by the finding of a central scotoma, and an optic neuritis may be mimicked. With compression however, the acuity continues to fall and the scotoma increases in size, breaking out to the periphery. If the compression is at the anterior angle of the chiasm, a small defect in the upper outer segment of the field of the other eye may be detectable [Figures 1.4 and 1.5 I(c)]. This results from the way some inferior nasal fibres cross from the other side and loop forward into the anatomical optic nerve at the front of the chiasm.

The hallmark of lesions at the chiasm is of a bitemporal defect, whether this is a complete hemianopia, upper or lower quadrant loss or central scotoma. Sometimes it may only be appreciated with a red target. If the chiasm is compressed from below (pituitary adenoma) upper quadrants may be affected first and show the greater loss. If the chiasm is affected from above (craniopharyngioma) bitemporal lower quadrant field loss

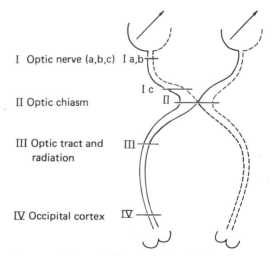

Figure 1.4 Schematic diagram of the visual pathway.

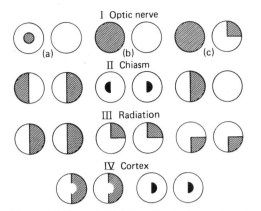

I Optic nerve

II Chiasm

III Radiation

IV Cortex

Figure 1.5 Visual field defects (for further explanation *see* text). Numbers refer to anatomical sites of responsible lesions in *Figure 1.4*.

predominates. Rarely lateral pressure on the chiasm (carotid aneurysm) produces a unilateral nasal field defect [Figure 1.5 II(c)]. Bitemporal scotomas can be caused if a pituitary tumour catches the central macular fibres which cross at the back of the chiasm.

Behind the chiasm, lesions in the tract and radiation alike produce a homonymous hemianopia. Tract lesions are rare, but important as they are usually due to middle cranial fossa tumours. They tend to be incongruous, the defect in the two eyes not matching exactly as fibres from comparable parts of the retina do not run together until after the relay in the lateral geniculate body. Radiation lesions are far more common and are usually due to vascular problems. The radiation sweeps laterally and posteriorly from the trigone of the lateral ventricle, which overlies the lateral geniculate relay, to reach the visual cortex in the occipital lobe. As it passes laterally and backwards it fans out, and may be affected in the parietal and temporal lobes. Parietal lesions affecting the upper fibres cause predominantly lower quadrantic defects. Temporal lobe lesions cause a predominantly upper quadrantanopia.

To understand lesions in the occipital lobe requires an understanding of the vascular supply of the visual cortex since nearly all lesions in this region are vascular. The banks of the calcarine fissure are supplied by the posterior cerebral artery. Its occlusion causes a hemianopia which may not affect the macula area,

since this is represented at the occipital pole which often has a dual blood supply also being reached by posterior parietal branches of the middle cerebral artery. By contrast patients sustaining a severe hypotensive crisis, e.g. after cardiac arrest, may awake with central field loss due to watershed infarction of the occipital poles at the vulnerable end of the supply of both the middle cerebral and posterior cerebral arteries.

Pupils

Pupil responses should be tested with an adequate bright light. Most ophthalmoscopes are inadequate for this purpose and tired batteries in small torches cause great confusion. Each eye should be tested in turn, and no eye drops should have been used.

Pupil size may be revealing (Table 1.5). Large pupils are normal in youth, and small pupils in old age. Amphetamines may cause large pupils, opiates small pupils. A large, slowly reacting pupil in a young female (Adie pupil) may be accompanied by loss of tendon reflexes. It causes alarm as some difficulty in focusing is experienced, especially at the time the abnormality develops. It is, however, a benign phenomenon. It is characterized by the slow though eventually normal range of pupil reaction to convergence and to light including delayed dilatation in the dark, and by denervation hypersensitivity to 2.5% methacholine drops. Acute glaucoma may be

Table 1.5 Pupillary abnormalities

Light reaction	Small pupil	Large pupil
Normal	Old age Horner's Pontine lesion	Young Anxiety
Impaired	Pilocarpine drops (for glaucoma) Opiates Argyll- Robertson	Atropine drops Amphetamine overdose Holmes-Adie Anoxia Brain death Brain stem stroke Carotid aneurysm (unilateral) Blind eye

accompanied by a large pupil. Anoxic brain damage causes bilateral dilated pupils.

A small pupil may be due to autonomic damage (Horner's syndrome) with a slight ptosis of the upper lid that is overcome during upgaze. There may or may not be loss of sweating on the face. A Horner's syndrome may develop from an intraocular lesion, from disease of the central nervous system, or more usually from damage to T1 sympathetic fibres in the neck (Pancoast's tumour, brachial plexus trauma, lymphadenopathy, carotid occlusions). If the cause is central, for example due to a medullary infarct, the pupil will still dilate to 1% hydroxyamphetamine, proof that the distal neurone is intact (Table 1.6). If the Horner's syndrome is due to a distal lesion this test is negative. The Horner's pupil fails to dilate to 10% cocaine. If congenital in origin it may be associated with a different coloured iris on that side. Iritis may cause a small pupil. Pontine disease, e.g. a pontine haemorrhage, can produce bilateral pin-point pupils which none the less react to light, albeit through a limited range that can be difficult to detect. Pupil responses are sluggish if acuity is poor due to retinal or optic nerve or chiasmatic damage. A difference in response when the light is shone obliquely from either side may be detectable with a lesion of the optic tract (thereby distinguishing it from a lesion in the optic radiation producing a similar field defect). This is an unreliable sign however, as the cornea and anterior chamber scatter the light path and frustrate the attempt to only illuminate one half of the retina. Pupil responses are lost after anoxic brain damage and in brain death.

A relatively reduced pupil reaction may be a useful sign of an old optic neuritis, thus helping to diagnose multiple sclerosis. To demonstrate this, the light is swung from one eye to the other. As the light shines into the affected 'bad' eye its pupil paradoxically dilates, losing more from the light leaving the good eye that was providing a strong consensual response than it gains from direct illumination through its own direct response carried by a defective optic nerve. This is the 'relative afferent pupillary defect' detected by the 'swinging light test'. Pupil responses are unaffected by opacities of the cornea, lens or vitreous, or by papilloedema.

Dilatation of one pupil follows impairment of the pupillomotor fibres in the third nerve. These are superficially placed in the nerve and are vulnerable to external pressure, as produced by an aneurysm on the internal carotid or posterior communicating artery, or from herniation of the temporal lobe onto the nerve between the brain stem and the free edge of the tentorium cerebelli, as occurs when there is a supratentorial mass lesion. In the latter case the patient's level of consciousness will be depressed. A third nerve palsy due to diabetes mellitus and vasculitis may spare the pupil.

The convergence reflex is observed as gaze is shifted from the distance to a near point. It is fully developed only if the convergence movement is adequate, and this depends on the patient being able to focus on the near object. This means that the test may have to be carried out with the patient wearing his glasses. Loss of light reflex with preservation of the convergence response occurs in syphilis (Argyll–Robertson pupil which is small and irregular), and with tumours and other lesions in the region of the pineal gland when the pupil is normal in shape and may be enlarged. Irregularity of the pupils is also seen with local inflammation (uveitis).

3rd, 4th and 6th nerves

These are examined collectively by observing eye movement which also tests the supranuclear pathways controlling horizontal and vertical gaze. Eye movements are generated in three ways (Figure 1.6), each of which can be

Table 1.6 Pupil responses in Horner's syndrome

	1%	1%
	Hydroxyamphetamine (tests viability postganglionic fibres)	Phenylephrine (detects denervation hypersensitivity)
Central	Dilates (as does normal)	Unaffected (as is normal)
Peripheral	Unaffected (normal dilates)	Dilates (more than normal)

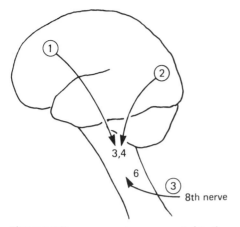

Figure 1.6 Eye movements are generated in three ways. 1 = Frontal; rapid voluntary movements. 2 = Occipital; slow following movements. 3 = Vestibular; reflex movements.

tested separately. Voluntary movements are generated in the frontal lobe, following or pursuit movements in the occipital region. Finally, movements occur in response to head movements due to vestibular reflexes. These can be elicited by rotating the head from side to side and up and down while asking the patient to fixate on a point straight ahead in space. The eyes roll in the opposite direction to maintain fixation. This 'doll's head' manoeuvre is the easiest way to test eye movements in the lightly unconscious patient **(see p. 66).**

When using a hand as a target for patients to follow whilst testing pursuit eye movements, the patient's head may have to be steadied by a finger on the chin, and it is important not to move the target too rapidly nor to hold it too close to the eyes. If the latter mistake is made convergence contaminates the following movements and they may not appear full. Other patients have spasm of convergence causing diplopia and apparent weakness of abduction. The clue that this is happening is that the pupils can be seen to constrict as they look to the side. In the elderly convergence and upgaze become restricted, so allowances must be made before deciding such movements are defective.

Some individuals have a tendency to divergence or convergence of the eyes which leads to confusion when testing. It is revealed by the cover test. The patient looks at a target such as the examiner's finger held directly in front of him. The examiner's other hand is interposed to obscure one of the patient's eyes and enforce fixation by the other. As the hand is removed the convergent or divergent position of the masked eye is briefly seen before it fixes on the target. Its lack of movement disorder is confirmed by a full range when tested monocularly. Such a latent squint may be a cause of double vision when it 'breaks down' because of some impairment of acuity or even a nonspecific debilitating illness or fatigue. To test convergence, the long-sighted patient must wear his glasses so that he can focus on the approaching target adequately. Loss of voluntary and following movements to one side may be due to a hemisphere lesion when head rolling will produce the otherwise absent horizontal gaze, or from a pontine lesion when all attempts to cause lateral gaze will fail. The rest position of the eyes when horizontal gaze to one side has been lost in a hemisphere lesion is to the side of the lesion; 'the eyes look at the lesion'. When a pontine lesion causes unilateral loss of horizontal gaze the eyes drift towards the intact side. The exception to this rule arises when an irritative frontal lobe lesion causes a seizure with head and/or eye turning to the opposite side.

Upgaze can be restricted in old age and in Parkinson's disease, but can also be an important sign of frontal lobe lesions or abnormality at the top of the brain stem.

Horizontal gaze requires the yoking together of the two eyes (Figure 1.7). Abduction of one eye, brought about by its 6th nerve nucleus in the pons near the lateral pontine gaze centre, needs to be accompanied by adduction of the other eye, a 3rd nerve function. Messages travel from the region of the lateral pontine gaze centre and 6th nerve nucleus to the opposite 3rd nerve in the medial longitudinal bundle. If this bundle is damaged, then horizontal gaze is no longer conjugate as the two eyes no longer move in concert. The abducting eye moves, though it shows the alternating slow and quick movements of nystagmus, whilst the adducting eye fails (Figure 1.8). Getting the patient to switch rapidly from a central to a lateral target may reveal the slow adduction. Such an

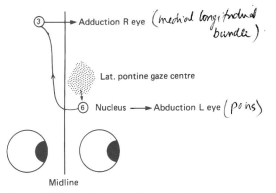

Figure 1.7 Normal horizontal gaze involves yoking together of the eyes through an interconnection between the 6th nerve nucleus of the abducting eye and the 3rd nerve nucleus of the contralateral adducting eye.

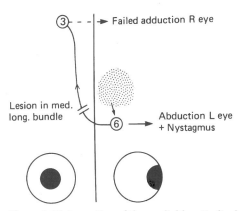

Figure 1.8 Interruption of the medial longitudinal bundle leads to nystagmus in the abducting eye (ataxic nystagmus) and defective adduction of the other eye (internuclear ophthalmoplegia), a common sign of brain stem involvement in multiple sclerosis.

'internuclear ophthalmoplegia' (the lesion is between or *inter* the nuclei) with 'ataxic' nystagmus is a common physical sign in multiple sclerosis and is evidence of an intrinsic brain stem lesion. When unilateral, and only seen on gaze to one side it may also be due to a vascular lesion. If there are no other features of central nervous system disease the possibility that a similar picture is due to myasthenia gravis should, however, be considered. Fatiguable ptosis, and great variability in the signs may be the clue to this rare 'pseudo'-internuclear ophthalmoplegia.

Individual lesions of 3rd, 4th and 6th cranial nerves cause simple paresis of ocular movements (Figure 1.9). A 6th nerve lesion causes isolated loss of abduction with horizontal diplopia, especially at a distance. At the near point, convergence is normal so the diplopia disappears. The usual cause is raised intracranial pressure, especially in children, and vascular damage in the elderly. The combination of a 6th nerve palsy and a hemiparesis suggests a pontine glioma in childhood, multiple sclerosis in the young adult and a pontine infarct in the elderly. A 4th nerve lesion causes difficulty in depressing the adducted eye, so the patients are at risk on stairs, the tread appearing double or blurred so they miss their footing. Ironically, head injury is the usual cause, as well as a possible consequence, of a 4th nerve palsy. Head tilt corrects the diplopia of a fourth nerve palsy. A mechanical problem with the trochlear can cause the same functional deficit again after trauma or in rheumatoid arthritis.

Complete 3rd nerve lesions cause paralysis of the lid (ptosis). The pupil is dilated and there is weakness of adduction, elevation, and depression of that eye. Spared abduction leads to lateral deviation of the eye at rest. The usual causes are external compression (when the pupil is affected) and microvascular damage, e.g. in diabetes mellitus when the peripherally lying pupillomotor fibres may be spared. The 3rd nerve palsy with a spared

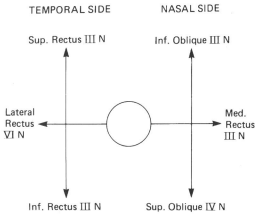

Figure 1.9 Eye muscles responsible for main movements of single eye. The recti elevate and depress the abducted eye, the obliques elevate and depress the adducted eye.

pupil is thus usually a 'medical' problem. If the pupil is affected the cause is usually 'surgical'. If the eye cannot be adducted because of a 3rd nerve palsy the function of the 4th nerve is difficult to assess. Attempts to look down and in will, however, reveal ocular rotation. Nuclear lesions of the 3rd nerve are rare but may cause added weakness of the superior rectus muscle of the other eye with bilateral ptosis. The ptosis of a third nerve palsy often causes mechanical difficulty with vision which contrasts with the much milder droop of the eyelid caused by a Horner's syndrome.

Combinations of lesions of the 3rd, 4th and 6th nerve, usually with sensory loss in the face because of concomitant 5th nerve damage, are encountered with lesions at the orbital fissure or in the cavernous sinus (e.g. aneurysms, meningioma, pituitary adenoma, pseudo tumour). If the cavernous sinus is thrombosed the picture is dominated by proptosis and oedema of the conjunctiva, and scleral injection. The combination of 3rd and 4th nerve palsies with a lesion of the 12th nerve is said to be characteristic of the effects of a nasopharyngeal carcinoma.

Lesions in the region of the pretectal plate, e.g. a pinealoma, cause loss of upgaze, lid retraction, impaired pupillary light reflexes and nystagmus on convergence. If the eyes are viewed from the side both globes appear to retract with each beat of the nystagmus (convergence–retraction nystagmus). This combination of signs is known as Parinaud's syndrome.

Ptosis

Ptosis can thus be due to Horner's syndrome, a third nerve palsy, ocular myopathy, myasthenia gravis, dystrophia myotonica, and brain stem disease.

Proptosis/exophthalmos

These terms both refer to forward displacement of the globe(s). The best way to detect such a shift is to observe the eyes from above and behind the patient's head. Exophthalmos refers to bilateral prominence of the eyes and is usually due to thyroid disease. There is swelling of intra-ocular muscles (visible on scanning). The eyelids are retracted, and lag behind on downgaze, exposing the sclera. There is often associated diplopia and restricted eye movement and if severe, exposure damage to the cornea.

Proptosis is used to describe unilateral protrusion of the globe. It can be due to a tumour, a granulomatous pseudotumour, a hamartomatous optic nerve 'glioma' in a young person, a mucocoele of the ethmoid sinus, a meningioma, or disease of the cavernous sinus. A haemangioblastoma may be suggested by an orbital bruit.

5th cranial nerve

Weakness of the masseter on one side is rarely seen. There is accompanying wasting, and a hollowing of one cheek may be detected. The muscle belly should be felt during forced jaw closure, and the central position of the chin observed during jaw opening (pterygoids also supplied by the 5th nerve). The jaw deviates towards the weak side. The pterygoids can also be checked by having the patient push his lower jaw to either side. The degree of overlap of lower teeth on the upper incisors during this test may reveal an asymmetry of range of lateral movement. Strength of jaw closure on the two sides can be assessed by pulling on a tongue depressor clamped by the patient's back teeth on either side. Bilateral weakness of the jaw is seen in myasthenia gravis and may lead to a characteristic sign in which the patient is seen to hold his chin up with his hand. The combination of bilateral ptosis and jaw support is particularly striking and enables a spot diagnosis to be made. Weakness is also seen in dystrophia myotonica.

The jaw jerk is important as it is the easiest 'tendon' reflex to elicit among the cranial nerves. It may be crucial in identifying the 'level' of a bilateral upper motor neurone lesion, although it may be risky to depend on this alone. If there are signs of increased tone and reflexes in upper and lower limbs, a normal jaw jerk will 'place' the lesion in the cervical cord. An equally enhanced jaw jerk will imply that the lesion is in the brain stem or hemispheres. The patient should be shown how to let his mouth sag open and a finger placed on the chin is then struck downwards by the tendon hammer.

Sensory disturbance in the face due to damage of the sensory roots of the 5th nerve is more common. There may be a small patch of numbness over the chin, for example with a skull base or mandibular metastasis, usually from carcinoma of the breast, or over the cheek from a lesion in the nasopharynx or orbital fissure. More widespread facial sensory disturbance may occur from more proximal 5th nerve involvement, e.g. in the cerebello-pontine angle, though the commonest tumour at this site, the acoustic neuroma, often only affects the corneal reflex. Central lesions may cause unilateral facial sensory loss as part of the hemianaesthesia of a thalamic or parietal lobe lesion. The sensory loss may be dissociated, with pain and temperature modalities being affected if the spinal nucleus and tract are affected, for example with a lateral medullary infarct. Hyperventilation causes parasthesiae in the circumoral region often associated with similar sensations or even tetany in the hands.

The corneal reflex may be tested by blowing gently on the cornea or by the touch of a wisp of cotton wool. Warn the patient what you intend before assaulting the sensitive cornea. The lower lid is held down while the patient looks up, making it easy to touch the lower cornea. Bilateral loss is rare, though some 'stoical' patients appear to have a depressed blink response to this stimulus. Unilateral depression or loss is far more likely to be important. If there is a concomitant 7th nerve lesion so that no blink can occur, the patient should be asked if they felt a sting when the cotton wool thread was touched against the lower cornea. The other eye should also be observed since the reflex involves both unilateral early and bilateral later responses. Rarely the corneal reflex is depressed by a deep lesion like a glioma or haematoma in the contralateral hemisphere. A twist of moistened cotton wool inserted up the nostril produces a reaction that may help decide if there is real sensory loss or not in the first division.

Isolated trigeminal neuropathy is rarely idiopathic, occasionally due to systemic sclerosis, and should always prompt a search for a skull base metastasis or nasopharyngeal tumour. 5th nerve involvement may be accompanied by ophthalmoplegia with orbital fissure lesions which usually cause proptosis, or from lesions in the cavernous sinus. The combination of painful trigeminal nerve damage and a 6th nerve palsy (Gradenigo's syndrome) arises from infection or tumour masses at the apex of the petrous temporal bone.

7th cranial nerve (Table 1.7)

The 7th nerve is responsible for movements of one side of the face. Movement of the forehead, looking surprised and frowning, eye closure, burying the eyelids, wrinkling the nose and pursing and pouting of the lips are all weakened by a lower motor neurone 7th nerve lesion. Spontaneous blinking may be asymmetrical, and the palpebral fissure widened. Patients need encouragement to close their eyes forcibly when this is being assessed and admonitions to pretend they are getting soap in their eyes may be necessary to get them to appreciate the kind of

Table 1.7 Facial weakness

Unilateral	Upper motor neurone (hemisphere)	e.g. stroke, tumour
	Nuclear (brain) stem)	Stroke (crossed hemiplegia), multiple sclerosis, pontine glioma
	Lower motor neurone	Bell's palsy, parotid tumour, acoustic neuroma
Bilateral	Upper motor neurone	Pseudobulbar palsy, bilateral strokes, motor neurone disease
	Lower motor neurone	Guillain-Barre, motor neurone disease, sarcoidosis
	Muscle	Facioscapulo-humeral dystrophy, dystrophia myotonica

movement wanted. If a full effort is made the eye rolls up behind the eyelid (Bell's phenomenon). The examiner should be prepared to press lightly with a finger laid along the line running vertically above the nose on the forehead to prevent movement on one side passively wrinkling the other brow, confusing assessment of local contraction. The examiner should use his fingers to see if he can overcome the patient's attempt to furrow his brow. Keeping the lips closed against the examiner who is trying to prize them apart may help reveal slight weakness of the orbicularis oris. To test the platysma the patient needs to be asked to protrude his chin and bare his teeth at the same time. The muscle then stands out. When the lower motor neurone weakness is profound and eye closure impossible the fact that the patient is trying to carry out the movement is revealed by the upward movement of the eye.

The commonest cause of a unilateral lower motor neurone weakness is the familiar Bell's palsy. In this benign condition, taste on the front of one side of the tongue may be affected as the chorda tympani runs with the facial nerve in its distal path. There may also be hyperacusis if the nerve to the stapedius is affected by a more proximally placed lesion of the facial nerve. Without damping of the ear drum loud sounds 'jar' and the patient complains of the harsh timbre of voices and telephone bells on the affected side. These phenomena help prove that the 7th nerve is damaged in its peripheral course rather than in the brain stem. In the latter case there is usually an accompanying 6th nerve palsy and long tracts are affected. Recovery from a Bell's palsy occurs in some 90% of cases but may be delayed and if regenerating axons reinnervate parts of the face different from their original connections, abnormal patterns of facial movement may result. Thus the eye may close on moving the lips. Spontaneous bursts of impulses may cause pulling movements of the face (hemifacial spasm). If the facial palsy is at onset incomplete, good recovery can be predicted.

Unilateral seventh nerve damage when not due to a Bell's palsy, can be due to herpes zoster, or skull fracture, and rarely to parotid malignancy, and other infections like otitis media, mumps, leprosy and Lyme disease. A lower motor neurone seventh nerve palsy with long tract signs suggests involvement of the fibres passing through the pons from the seventh nerve nucleus. This may occur with a pontine glioma, or in multiple sclerosis.

Bilateral seventh nerve palsies occur in Guillain–Barré, sarcoidosis, malignant meningitis and Lyme disease. Other cause of bilateral facial weakness include myasthenia gravis, dystrophica myotonica, polymyositis, and muscular dystrophy. Such patients' attempts to smile look more like a snarl.

Weakness restricted to a small area of the face may be due to a lesion in the parotid bed, and this may be the way a parotid tumour's aggressive behaviour comes to light. The lower corner of the mouth may droop from traumatic damage to a branch of the nerve, after carotid endarterectomy, or other neck surgery.

Supranuclear (upper motor neurone) weakness of the face spares the forehead, and eye closure is not as weak as the lower face. This is due to bilateral 'representation' of the forehead in the motor cortex. A dramatic confirmation of this is seen in rare cases of focal epilepsy in which both sides of the forehead convulse along with one side of the lower face. Greater weakness of the *lower* face is thus seen in upper motor neurone involvement, weakness of the *upper* face implying a lower motor neurone lesion. These distinctions can be difficult with a facial palsy of recent onset. Emotional movements, for example during laughing, are as affected as voluntary movements by facial nerve damage or thalamic / brain stem lesions but may be spared with cortical lesions. The patient should be induced to smile or laugh to check this. A minimal upper motor neurone weakness may be detected by an asymmetry of burying the eyelashes or of the 'O' made by the widely opened mouth. Bilateral upper motor neurone weakness is usually accompanied by a spastic dysarthria, and brisk jaw and gag reflexes. If the pursed lips are tapped a brisk pout reflex may result.

Taste on the front of the tongue travels to the geniculate ganglion in fibres that accompany the seventh nerve. Loss of taste is more usually due to systemic factors like drugs, hepatitis, malignancy or systemic sclerosis, rather than neurological illness.

8th cranial nerve

Both auditory and vestibular branches can be tested. Hearing can be assessed at the bedside by the simple expedient of seeing whether the patient can hear a whispered voice at 2 feet (60 cm). While testing, a fingertip should be vibrated in the other external auditory meatus to mask it, lest unilateral hearing loss be missed owing to the other ear hearing the voice. The examiner's face should be out of sight to prevent lip reading. If hearing loss is demonstrated by this screening test or suspected, proper audiometry should be carried out. However, the important distinction between conductive hearing loss due to disease of the middle ear and hearing loss due to a lesion of the cochlea or auditory nerve can be made with a tuning fork. Normally, thanks to the amplification produced by the middle ear, a fork (512 Hz) held at the external auditory meatus sounds louder than when its base plate is pressed onto the mastoid process. The fork should be set in motion by a blow on the hand or knee. If struck against a table unwanted harmonics are produced. If the hearing loss is 'conductive' from middle-ear disease then the fork heard through bone sounds louder than when it is heard through the air. The normal, air louder than bone, pattern is retained for cochlear or nerve hearing loss. Tuning fork tests are not always reliable, however, and audiometry is required if hearing loss is detected or suspected.

Audiometry confirms the presence of defective hearing, quantitates it and defines the frequency spectrum affected. Nerve hearing loss usually affects high frequencies first; conductive hearing loss usually starts with low frequencies. High-tone hearing loss is also characteristic of that produced by exposure to loud noises. The audiometric testing also compares air and bone conduction. Two important phenomena are sought by special techniques. 'Tone decay' refers to the way a tone has to be made louder to maintain its subjective loudness as the hearing fatigues and is marked with 8th nerve lesions including acoustic neuromas. 'Loudness recruitment' refers to the subjective normality of loud sounds in an ear that fails to hear quieter sounds, when compared with its partner. This phenomenon is a good clue to a lesion in the cochlea such as Ménière's disease.

Nystagmus

The vestibular part of the nerve is assessed by a search for spontaneous nystagmus, and tests of induced nystagmus.

Nystagmus is a to and fro movement of the eyes which is usually due to a defect of control of eye movement emanating from the labyrinths or their central brain stem connections. Rarely, a pendular movement of the eyes of equal velocity in both directions is seen owing to poor vision from early life. This ocular nystagmus may be seen with albinism and congenital cataracts, for example. Rarely, something similar is seen in multiple sclerosis. The nystagmus due to labyrinthine or brain stem disease has an alternating slow drift, usually back off the eccentric target, and quick movement outwards, back on to the target. Weakness of gaze must not be assumed to be its basic cause but it does 'look' as though the eyes are finding it difficult to maintain a deviation and slowly move back towards a central rest position. The quick movement follows to restore the desired position. This description is given solely as an aide-memoire. The nystagmus seen through an ophthalmoscope beats in the opposite direction from the movement of the front of the eye.

Testing for nystagmus requires care. Normals may develop a few beats of nystagmus at extremes of gaze so the target (usually the examiner's finger) should not go beyond the point of bilateral fixation and preferably only 30° from the straight-ahead position. If nystagmus is seen at full gaze, bringing the target back 10° will reveal whether it must be considered pathological, because it persists in this position.

Nystagmus from a labyrinthine lesion is distinguishable from that due to a brain-stem lesion by simple bedside observation (Table 1.8). That due to a peripheral lesion is temporary, horizontal, conjugate, unidirectional, and accompanied by vertigo. It may increase while

Table 1.8 Origin of nystagmus

	Peripheral (labyrinth)	Central (brain stem)
Duration	Short, e.g. 3 weeks	Prolonged, often years
Vertigo	Linked	Dissociated (may be none)
Direction	Unilateral Horizontal Conjugate	Multidirectional Vertical Can be dysconjugate
Effect of loss fixation (Frenzel's glasses)	Increased	Not increased

being observed through an ophthalmoscope if the other eye is closed. That of brain-stem origin is often multi-directional, may persist for months or years and may be dissociated from any symptoms. Vertical nystagmus is always central (i.e. brain stem) in origin and therefore pathological. The commonest cause of symmetrical horizontal nystagmus quick-phase to the right on looking to the right, quick-phase to the left on looking to the left, is drug effect. Hypnotics, sedative tranquillizers, and anti-epileptic drugs are most likely to cause such nystagmus. Ototoxic drugs like streptomycin, kanamicin and gentamicin by contrast produce gradual bilateral peripheral labyrinthine failure with no spontaneous

nystagmus, but ataxia on attempting to stand and walk. The patients may also complain that the visual world bounces as they walk (oscillopsia). Such illusory movement is less common with central lesions. Special types of nystagmus, most reflecting central lesions, may have further localizing value (Table 1.9). Complex combinations of ophthalmoplegia and nystagmus are seen in myasthenia gravis, and with ataxia in Wernicke's encephalopathy.

Induced nystagmus

Caloric stimulation mimics rotation of the head by inducing convection currents in the semicircular canal. Warm (44°C) or cool (30°C,) water is run into the external auditory meatus for 40 seconds with the patient lying on a couch with 30° head-up tilt. This places the horizontal semicircular canal in the vertical plane, and ensures its maximal stimulation. Convection currents in the endolymph are set up by the temperature change and these stimulate the hair cells mimicking the effects of rotation. Nystagmus away from the ear with cool water and towards the ear with warm water is timed (mnemonic: cold opposite warm same = COWS) (Figure 1.10). No nystagmus is seen if a labyrinth is dead, a so-called 'canal paresis'. A tendency for nystagmus to be more developed to one direction

Table 1.9 Types of nystagmus

Type	Appearance	Lesion
Rotary	Mixed rotary and horizontal	Labyrinth
	Pure	Vestibular nuclei
Ataxic	Greater in abducting eye	Medial longitudinal bundle
Vertical	1. Up beating	Brain stem or cerebellum
	2. Down beating	Craniocervical junction Cerebellar degeneration
See-saw	One up one down with rotary component	Para-pituitary region
Positioning	1. With delay, adapts, fatigues, with vertigo	Posterior canal
	2. Persists, many positions, often no vertigo	Posterior fossa
Alternating	To one side, then reverses	Unknown
Congenital	Pendular at rest, jerk to side	Unknown
Pendular	Same velocity each phase	Poor acuity since childhood
Jelly	Very rapid oscillation	Brain stem (multiple sclerosis)
Rebound	On return to centre	Cerebellum
Convergence-retraction	Seen from side	Tectal plate (Parinaud's syndrome)
Bruns	Slow coarse to one side, rapid fine to other	Cerebellopontine angle
Opsoclonus	Chaotic jerks, causing impaired vision	Viral encephalitis, neuroblastoma

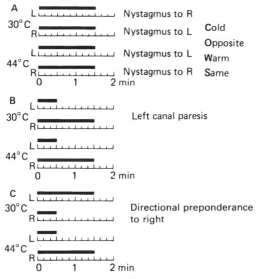

A
30°C
L ▬▬▬▬▬ Nystagmus to R
R ▭▭▭▭▭ Nystagmus to L   Cold
                          Opposite
44°C
L ▬▬▬▬ Nystagmus to L   Warm
R ▭▭▭▭▭ Nystagmus to R   Same
0   1   2 min

B
30°C
L ▬
R ▬▬▬▬   Left canal paresis
44°C
L ▬
R ▬▬▬
0   1   2 min

C
30°C
L ▭▭▭▭▭   Directional preponderance
R ▬   to right
44°C
L ▭▭▭▭
R ▬▬▬
0   1   2 min

Figure 1.10 Caloric test. Induced caloric nystagmus may reveal abnormalities of impaired responsiveness (canal paresis), or a tendency to asymmetry (directional preponderance) in both peripheral and central lesions of the 8th nerve system.

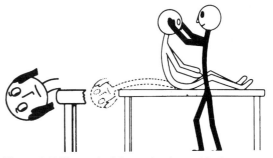

Figure 1.11 The method for testing for positioning nystagmus. (After Dix, with permission.)

whether induced by cold water in one ear, or warm water in the other is called 'directional preponderance'. This abnormal pattern of caloric responsiveness may be seen with peripheral or central abnormalities. The combination of sensorineural hearing loss with tone decay and canal paresis is characteristic of an acoustic neuroma whilst sensorineural hearing loss with loudness recruitment and canal paresis or directional preponderance suggests Ménière's disease. Directional preponderance is towards the side of a cerebellar lesion but away from the side of a vestibular one.

The utricle/posterior canal can be tested by a search for positioning nystagmus (Figure 1.11). The patient sits on a flat couch and is then asked to lie back with his head turned to one side, hanging over the end of the bed. This tests the undermost ear. If it is faulty, nystagmus beating towards the floor develops after a brief latent interval only to fatigue away. Repetition of the positioning causes less nystagmus. This type of nystagmus is usually accompanied by vertigo and is a common cause of dizziness after head injury and with labyrinthine lesions of all sorts, though it may

occur 'out of the blue' (benign positioning vertigo). If positioning provokes a lasting nystagmus with no delay, which does not adapt on repetition and is seen whether the head is to the left or to the right, a central cause is likely. In practice such patients commonly have cerebellar degeneration, multiple sclerosis, or a posterior fossa metastasis.

Optokinetic nystagmus (OKN)

If the vertical stripes on a rotating drum are watched by an alert co-operative subject, following movements alternate with quick eye movements back onto the next target (next stripe). This phenomenon is seen in individuals watching the passing telegraph poles from the seat of a moving train and is physiological. Its development requires intact fixation (so it can be used to test visual acuity in the illiterate and young) and a connection through the parietal area between the visual cortex and the frontal areas for rapid eye movements. An asymmetry of the response, commonly a loss when the drum rotates one way, can therefore be a sign of a parietal lobe lesion. It does not depend on the presence of a hemianopia and is worth seeking in a possible hemisphere lesion even when there are no visual symptoms and no field defects. It may also help locate the lesion causing a hemianopia. OKN may be normal with an occipital infarct (posterior cerebral artery territory) but affected with a hemianopia owing to a deep lesion in the radiation (more likely to be in the middle cerebral artery territory). An asymmetrical response can also be seen with cerebellar and brain-stem disease. The test is normal in the presence of labyrinthine disease, which makes it valuable for screening in patients with vertigo, etc. It is lost in cortical blindness.

In the presence of congenital nystagmus, the optokinetic response may occur in the opposite direction to normal.

9th and 10th cranial nerves

Routine testing of the gag reflex, palatal and pharyngeal movement and sensation and movement of the vocal cords is rarely necessary, but is obviously crucial when symptoms suggest bulbar problems. Touching the pharynx with an orange stick tests pharyngeal sensation (9th cranial nerve) and the gag reflex (9th and 10th). Occasionally normal individuals appear to be stoically unaffected by the stimulus despite feeling it normally. On phonation the palate should rise in the midline (10th nerve). Unilateral paralysis causes peaking of one side only. Bilateral paresis causes nasal regurgitation of food, a nasal speech and the palate fails to move on phonation, e.g. when saying 'Ah' or in the gag reflex. Nasal escape during phonation can be checked by placing a cold surface (hand mirror) at the nasal orifice while the patient says 'pa pa pa'. Misting over of the surface can be seen with each utterance.

Vocal cord weakness (10th nerve) may be tested crudely by listening to the patient cough. Approximation of the cords is needed for the normal explosive onset of the sound. With bilateral cord paralysis the cough is said to be 'bovine' though not all students have listened to a cow cough! Bilateral cord paralysis causes loss of voice, an inability to cough, and stridor. A mirror examination should be carried out if there is any question of any disturbance of lower cranial nerves, to visualize the cords and simultaneously to exclude a nasopharyngeal tumour as a cause. Biopsy of the posterior nasopharyngeal space may be revealing even when the mirror examination appears normal. Lesions at the jugular foramen like a glomus tumour, or malignant lymph node may cause combinations of lower cranial nerve palsies. Upper motor neurone weakness of the palate is distinguished by the briskness of the gag reflex in contrast to the paresis of voluntary movement in phonation, and it is usually accompanied by a spastic tongue and a brisk jaw jerk (pseudobulbar palsy).

11th cranial nerve

The function of this nerve is checked by testing the power of the sternomastoid and trapezius muscles. The sternomastoid is a prime mover in the act of rotation of the head to the other side when the power of movement can be gauged by a hand on the opposite side of the jaw, and the bulk seen and felt. The sternomastoid is connected to its ipsilateral hemisphere as movement of the head to the right and the right-sided limbs are all represented in the left hemisphere and head rotation to the right is carried out by the left sternomastoid. Upper motor neurone lesions thus involve weakness of the sternomastoid muscle contralateral to the hemiparesis they cause, and weakness and delay of shoulder shrugging (trapezius) on the side of the hemiparesis. Testing shoulder shrugging can be useful when lack of facial weakness leaves the examiner unsure whether a hemiparesis is due to disease of the brain or cervical cord. Normal shrugging would suggest a cord lesion below the supply to the trapezius (C1–5).

Bilateral weakness of the sternomastoid and other neck muscles is common in myopathies (polymyositis, scleroderma), motor neurone disease and myasthenia gravis. Bilateral wasting is also characteristic of dystrophia myotonica. Weakness of trapezii makes the head drop forwards. Weakness of sternomastoids make it difficult to lift the head off the pillow without using a throwing action.

The trapezius is responsible for shrugging of the shoulders and plays a part in anchoring the scapula to the thorax. Slight winging and rotation of the scapula at rest occurs with selective loss of the trapezius. The top of the scapula moves down and out, the bottom up and in. The mild separation of the scapula away from the chest wall is increased by abduction of the arm, and reduced by elevation of the arm in front of the patient (flexion).

Severe winging develops from damage to the long nerve of Bell with weakness of the serratus anterior. The separation is reduced by abduction and much increased by flexion of the arm with an attempt to push forwards (Figure 1.12).

Unilateral 11th nerve lesions are rare except with trauma to the neck often due to biopsy or surgical dissection of malignant lymph nodes, or with tumours at the jugular foramen such as a glomus jugulare.

12th cranial nerve

This is solely responsible for the musculature of the tongue. Isolated damage to one hypoglossal nerve causes unilateral wasting of the tongue and the tongue deviates towards the weak side on protrusion due to the unopposed action of the muscle on the normal side. The strength of the two sides can also be compared by getting the patient to push his tongue into either cheek, and opposing the movement with a finger on the outside. A unilateral 12th nerve palsy is often due to malignant meningitis or to a tumour at the foramen magnum or to a skull base fracture. Manipulation of food in the mouth and swallowing are disturbed.

A unilateral upper motor neurone disturbance produces little or no difficulty with tongue movements but diction and swallowing may be transiently mildly impaired, and tongue protrusion may be eccentric in the acute stages after a stroke. Bilateral lower motor neurone involvement (bulbar palsy–bulb = medulla) occurs in motor neurone disease (MND) and with brain-stem gliomas, the Arnold–Chiari malformation or malignant meningitis when a small wasted tongue may eventually become immobile. It may show a fine rippling movement on its surface due to contraction of individual motor units — fasciculation. These may occur in the normal subject if the muscle is contracted, so must be sought with the tongue at rest in the mouth and not protruded.

Bilateral upper motor neurone involvement may occur after bilateral strokes or with multiple sclerosis or MND (pseudobulbar palsy). Now there is a small spastic non-fasciculating tongue that is stiff to move and causes a thick speech. If the patient is asked to protrude the tongue and wriggle it from side to side, the movement is slowed. Some people have difficulty with lateral movements of the tongue and it can be more revealing to ask for the tongue to be put in and out quickly. In these circumstances the jaw jerk is brisk, emotional facial movements and tearing may be exaggerated and the gag reflex is brisker than normal.

Combinations of lower cranial nerve lesions, if all on one side, usually prove to be due to a skull base tumour, often metastatic (Table 1.10). Bilateral lower cranial nerve palsies can be due to malignant meningitis, sarcoidosis or a kind of Guillain–Barré polyneuritis.

Intrinsic brain-stem lesions may cause a combination of cranial nerve signs (as evidence of the location of the problem) together with weakness or sensory loss in the limbs due to involvement of the long tracts passing through the brain stem, or ataxia due to disturbance in the cerebellar peduncles or area of the red nucleus (Table 1.11).

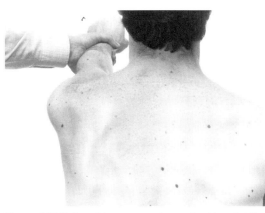

Figure 1.12 If the subject presses forward with a rigidly extended arm, the ability of the serratus anterior to hold the scapula to the chest wall is tested. If weak, the scapula 'wings' (C5–7).

Further reading

MAYO CLINIC DEPARTMENT OF NEUROLOGY (1991) *Clinical Examination in Neurology*, 6th edn. Mosby Year Book, St Louis.

Table 1.10 Cranial nerve syndromes

Site	Nerves	Cause
Carvernous sinus	3, 4, 5^I, 6 ± proptosis	Aneurysm, mass from sinus or granuloma
Apex petrous temporal bone	5, 6	Metastasis
Cerebellopontine angle	5, 7, 8 ± 9	Acoustic neuroma, meningioma, epidermoid, aneurysm
Jugular foramen	9, 10, 11	Tumour, aneurysm, lymph node
Meninges	Bilateral combinations	Malignant meningitis, sarcoidosis, tuberculosis

Table 1.11 Brain-stem syndromes

Site of lesion	Structures affected	Clinical picture
Tectal plate	Posterior commissure	Loss of upgaze, fixed pupils, convergence nystagmus
Paramedian midbrain	3rd nerve nucleus ± corticospinal tract ± medial lemniscus ± red nucleus	3rd nerve palsy ± crossed hemiplegia or hemianaesthesia ± coarse tremor
Paramedian pons	6th and 7th nerve nuclei + corticospinal tract	6th and 7th nerve palsy and crossed hemiplegia
Cerebellopontine angle	8th nerve, 5th nerve, 6th and 7th nerves, vestibular nuclei, cerebellar hemisphere, corticospinal tract	Ipsilateral deafness, loss corneal reflex, nystagmus, 6th and 7th nerve weaknesses, ataxia, contralateral hemiparesis
Lateral medulla	Spinal nucleus of 5th, 9th, 10th and 11th nerve nuclei, spinothalamic, spinocerebellar and also cerebellar tracts	Ipsilateral 5th, 9th, 10th, 11th nerve lesions, Horner's syndrome and ataxia, contralateral pain and temperature loss
Foramen magnum	Cerebellar tonsils, compression dorsal columns, corticospinal tracts	Downbeat nystagmus, ataxia limbs, bilateral pyramidal signs, joint position sense loss (hands > feet)

BICKERSTAFF, E. (1980) *Neurological Examination in Clinical Practice*, 4th edn. Blackwell Scientific Publications, Oxford.

GLASER, J.S. (1990) *Neuro-ophthalmology*. Lippincott, Philadelphia

HAYMAKER, W. (1969) *Bing's Local Diagnosis in Neurological Disease*. C.V. Mosby, St. Louis.

HAWKES, C.H. (1993) Using 'smart handles' to make a rapid neurological diagnosis. *Hospital Update*, **19**, 333–351.

Motor system

The assessment of the motor system begins as soon as the patient enters the room. The way he walks, swings his arms, sits, undoes coat buttons and undresses for the examination provides much information about motor skills and speed. These initial observations have the additional advantage of being completed before the patient is aware that he is being examined.

Simple observation and palpation of muscle bulk is the first move. Muscle wasting develops rapidly with damage to anterior horn cells, e.g. in motor neurone disease, or axons (root, plexus or peripheral nerve lesions). Difficulties arise in the elderly in whom small hand muscles become thinner without pathological significance. The distinguishing feature is the relative preservation of power if the changes are simply age related. Muscle wasting also occurs around diseased joints though reflexes are not affected. The quadriceps, for example, loses bulk with osteoarthritis of the knee and hand muscles become thinner in rheumatoid arthritis. EMG studies may be needed in the latter case to distinguish between disuse atrophy and neuropathy which can complicate rheumatoid arthritis. Loss of bulk also occurs in wasting diseases like cancer, tuberculosis, malabsorption, and AIDS. Power is relatively well preserved however, and contrasts with the very thin spindly limbs. Mild asymmetries of muscle bulk should also be interpreted with caution as asymmetrical development is not uncommon. A hemiparesis developing in infancy or present from birth as well as affecting the degree of muscle development is revealed by the asymmetrical limb growth. Hands and feet should be inspected side by side for evidence of smallness of digits or foot size on the affected side. Hypertrophy of muscles occurs with athletic training and in the rare congenital myotonia. Pseudohypertrophy occurs in some genetically determined muscular dystrophies. The weak muscle is of larger bulk owing to an increase in connective tissue and fat, not muscle. Clawing of the hands and feet (pes cavus) is seen in some hereditary neuropathies.

Fasciculation in limb muscles as in the tongue implies a lower motor neurone lesion. Telltale rippling of the affected muscle must be sought in the resting state. Fasciculation after contraction is not necessarily pathological so it is a mistake to look for it after testing power. Muscles should not be percussed to see if they fasciculate, since only spontaneous fasciculation is a reliable sign of disease. Fasciculation in the calves can also be a benign phenomenon and affects many individuals, especially after exercise. Generalized fasciculation is often due to motor neurone disease when it is accompanied by muscular wasting and weakness, but is occasionally hereditary. Fasciculation may alternatively be restricted to one or two muscles. Thus it might be seen in the deltoid and biceps with a C5 root lesion due to cervical spondylosis.

While observing the limbs at rest for bulk and for fasciculation, note is taken of any deformities or postural abnormalities. Thus the hemiplegic leg lies extended and externally rotated.

The patient should be asked to hold their arms outstretched in front of them at shoulder height, with fingers horizontal. A wrist drop is characteristic of a radial nerve palsy. Droop of an individual finger is more likely to be due to motor neurone disease because of patchy loss of anterior horn cells. Involuntary separation of fingers due to weakness of adduction can be a sign of cervical myelopathy, or an ulnar nerve lesion if it only affects the little finger. Drift of the arm when the eyes are closed can be due to sensory loss (definitely the cause if the drift is upwards) or motor loss. The separated fingers in this position may reveal tremor or other involuntary movements not seen at rest. If the patient is then asked to rotate the hands palm up and hold them so whilst again closing their eyes a passive rolling inturning of one hand suggests an early upper motor neurone lesion affecting that side.

Increased tone may be suggested by a flexed posture of the arm, or by the puppet-like stiffness of the legs whilst walking. The response of the limbs to passive movements is the formal test of 'tone'. The resistance felt is partly due to the stiffness of joints, ligaments, etc., but partly due to the stretch reflex provoked in the main limb muscles. The assessment of tone (and reflexes) needs to be carried out in a relaxed warm subject. Spasticity due to hemisphere, brain-stem or spinal cord disease is best felt in the upper limb as a catch in passive stretch of the biceps as the elbow is extended and of the forearm pronators as the hand is held and the forearm supinated. Different speeds of movement have to be tried, as some may be more revealing than others. In the leg, alternating flexion and extension of the knee to look for an abnormal resistance to passive stretch of the quadriceps and hamstring muscles is usually frustrated by the patient immediately joining in, voluntarily flexing and extending the knee to 'help' the examiner, or immediately transforming the leg into a rigid pole. It is more useful to flick the knee in the air a few inches off the couch with a hand held under the popliteal fossa, whilst distracting the patient by conversation. In a limb of normal tone the heel stays on the couch and slides up and then down again as the leg falls back. If there is an enhanced stretch reflex in the quadriceps the jerk takes the heel off the bed where it hangs briefly before falling back. If increased 'spastic' resistance is felt at a joint, that resistance may collapse as the movement nears the end of its range (the clasp-knife reaction). Manipulating the legs of a patient with severe spasticity may provoke a slow extensor or flexor spasm in which the legs stiffen or draw up involuntarily. Similar spasms may occur spontaneously or be aggravated by sensory input from a bedsore or an infected bladder. These movements are a feature of spinal cord disease. A more diffuse increase in the tone in antagonists may be felt in the presence of frontal lobe lesions. This phenomenon (gegenhalten) feels as though the patient is deliberately counter-acting all imposed movements.

Another kind of resistance may be felt in patients with extrapyramidal diseases like Parkinson's disease. The limb feels like a piece of lead pipe which is equally stiff to bend in each direction and throughout the range of movement. It is best felt at the wrist during passive flexion and extension induced by holding the tips of the fingers. Again a spectrum of speed and range of induced movement helps to reveal any abnormality. This rigidity may be enhanced and thereby made easier to detect by the simple strategy of having the patient exercise the other arm. If the patient also has tremor, this may be detected as a regular interruption in the resistance to stretch — so-called cogwheel rigidity. Subtle increase in proximal muscle tone of this type may be detected by rocking the standing patient's shoulders to and fro with the examiner's hands on the front of the patient's shoulders. The flailing of the normal relaxed limb is replaced by a stiff movement en-bloc.

Reduced tone (hypotonia) occurs in cerebellar disease but is difficult to 'feel'. It may be suggested by hypermobility of joints or the tendency of a limb to oscillate after eliciting a tendon jerk. Thus if the patient sits on the side of the couch and the knee jerk is elicited, the lower leg may sway to and fro for several seconds (pendular knee jerk).

Reflexes

Abrupt muscle stretch by a brief blow to its tendon provokes a segmental reflex discharge of anterior horn cells with a resulting twitch contraction of the same muscle that can be seen and felt. Its vigour can be assessed by the size of the visible twitch and by any movement of the limb. A blow to the limb by a tendon hammer causes a shock wave through the limb and may elicit reflex contraction of another muscle whose tendon was not directly struck if its reflex arc is in a sufficiently excitable state. These monosynaptic reflexes are

very useful for testing the integrity of the arc (spindle — peripheral nerve — sensory root — dorsal root ganglion cell — anterior horn cell — motor root — peripheral nerve) and for assessing the balance of descending influences in the cord which reflect central abnormalities (enhanced reflexes from so-called upper motor neurone lesions in disease of the brain or cord).

Normally the jaw jerk, brachioradialis, biceps, triceps, knee and ankle tendon jerks (Table 1.12) should be sought plus the superficial reflexes produced by scratching the anterior abdominal wall and plantar surface of the foot. The muscle to be tested needs to be relaxed but under a degree of stretch. Thus it is normal to test the triceps, biceps, brachioradialis, knee and ankle jerks when their joints are flexed to 90°. The leg needs to be placed in the breast-stroke position for the ankle jerk, or the patient should kneel on a chair. If no reflex is obtained despite adequate co-operation in the form of relaxation, attempts should be made to enhance it. To this end, the patient forcibly contracts some other muscle groups. For example, while testing the reflexes of one arm the other hand may squeeze some convenient object such as the battery holder of an ophthalmoscope or make a tight fist and or clench his teeth. Whilst testing knee and ankle jerks, the flexed fingers of the two hands can be pulled against each other. The blow to the tendon should fall immediately after the reinforcing movement is started.

The commonest cause of loss of reflexes is poor technique with a clumsy blow with a hard hammer, off centre, to the tendon of a muscle held tight by a frightened patient.

Table 1.12 Reflexes

Cranial nerves	Jaw	5th cranial nerve
Upper limbs	Biceps	C5, 6
	Brachioradialis	C6
	Triceps	C7
	Finger flexion	C8
Trunk	Abdominal	T7-T12
	Cremaster	L1
Lower limbs	Knee	L3, 4
	Hamstring	L5, S1
	Ankle	(L5) S1
Sphincters	Bulbocavernosus	S3, 4, 5
	Anal	S4, 5

There is no loss of face in palpating for the tendon (especially that below the patella in an obese subject) before testing its reflex. True loss of reflex despite reinforcement implies interruption of the reflex arc and is, therefore, seen with root lesions and with peripheral nerve lesions. Loss of reflexes may also occur with advanced myopathies. A lost reflex can be heard as well as seen and felt, as its absence damps the blow of the tendon hammer more than usual, producing a dull 'thud'. Loss of both ankle jerks may occur in old age, but otherwise suggests peripheral neuropathy. Loss of a single ankle jerk is commonly due to the root damage of a prolapsed intervertebral disc. Loss of the biceps and brachioradialis reflex may be seen with C5–6 root lesions. If the cause is something like a disc, the cord may also be affected and the triceps (C7) and finger (C8) jerks brisker than normal. This may mean that a blow to the biceps tendon produces extension of the elbow by a triceps jerk, and a blow to the brachioradialis tendon produces finger flexion instead of elbow flexion. Such 'inversion' of these reflexes is pathognomic of a lesion at C5–6 at cord level, e.g. due to cervical spondylosis.

Enhanced reflexes may be due to nervousness, or thyrotoxicosis, when tone and power will be normal and the abdominal and plantar responses normal. In association with any of these other signs, however, they imply a lesion of the brain or spinal cord disinhibiting the local reflex arc. Very brisk reflexes in the legs may be considered evidence of abnormality if the reflexes of the upper limbs are normal, so excluding simple tension as a cause. Brisk reflexes in the fingers may occur in the normal; their asymmetry is a more useful sign of abnormality. To test for asymmetry in brisk reflexes, the tap on the tendon should be scaled down. However, if the only abnormality in a detailed neurological examination is reflex asymmetry, care should be taken not to over interpret this finding — it may prove to be illusory. The relaxation phase of tendon reflexes may be prolonged in hypothyroidism, hypothermia and with amyloidosis.

A downward tap on the chin when the jaw is allowed to fall half open may elicit a reflex in the masseter muscles. This jaw jerk is not elicited in all normals so care needs to be taken

in interpreting it. Its absence when there are brisk limb reflexes and other signs of upper motor neurone changes in the limbs is useful in suggesting that the causative lesion is below the level of the 5th nerve in the brain stem and probably in the high cervical cord. Bilateral hemiparesis (pseudo-bulbar palsy) from vascular disease characteristically causes a pathologically brisk jaw jerk as well as brisk reflexes in the limbs. Some primitive reflexes reappear in this context, a stroke across the palm may make the chin twitch (the palmo–mental reflex) and a tap on the lip may cause a pursing movement (pout reflex). These reflexes may be elicitable in normal subjects especially in old age, but in young and middle-aged subjects they can suggest upper motor neurone disturbance at hemisphere level and are often associated with a diffuse disease process.

A rapid shortening of a muscle may induce a repetitive oscillating contraction called clonus. This is most readily seen at the ankle when, with the knee flexed, the foot is suddenly dorsiflexed by the examiner's hand, which maintains pressure on the sole of the forefoot. A few beats (fewer than five) of the repetitive reflex may be seen in nervous individuals but persisting clonus implies pathologically enhanced reflexes. A sharp downward displacement of the patella by the examiner's open hand (forming a V between thumb and closed fingers astride the top edge of the patella) may cause patella clonus and similar movement may be rarely elicited in the flexors of the fingers or in supination of the forearm.

The superficial abdominal reflexes are elicited by scratching the anterior abdominal wall from the flank towards the midline parallel to the line of dermatomal strips slanting downwards as they come anteriorly. The reflexes are lost with upper motor neurone lesions above the level of about D6 or segmentally at the level of lower thoracic cord lesions. They are often but not universally lost early in the course of multiple sclerosis, but late in motor neurone disease. Unfortunately they are also lost in old age, after multiple pregnancies or abdominal operations, in gross obesity and if the patient tenses his abdominal wall. To be sure a reflex is missing, it must have been sought using the scratch of a pin, and the stimulus timed to coincide with relaxation at the end of expiration. Fatiguing the reflex by repetition may reveal an asymmetry in an early unilateral upper motor neurone lesion. A similar stroke of the top of the inner thigh will produce reflex contraction of the cremaster with ascent of the testicle on one side. This reflex is also lost with upper motor neurone lesions. It also tests the integrity of the L1 and L2 reflex arc so can be lost unilaterally with a root lesion.

The plantar response is a complicated reflex action to a noxious stimulus on the lateral margin of the sole of the foot. After infancy the normal response is of flexion of the big toe. In the presence of an upper motor neurone lesion the knee flexes, the toes fan and the big toe dorsiflexes slowly. This 'extensor' response is valuable proof of abnormality and of a cord or intracranial lesion but it can be difficult to assess. A nervous subject may withdraw the foot when the sole is scraped, obscuring the response. The first movement of the big toe is likely to be the reflex one when withdrawal occurs and is therefore the one to note. If, when the patient is ticklish, the plantar stimulation produces movement of the whole leg, it may help to elicit the reflex in other ways. A very laterally placed stimulus on the edge of the foot rather than on the sole (Chaddock's sign) may not prove so distressing to the patient. The thumb and index finger may be run firmly down the edge of the tibia (Oppenheim's sign), the little toe may be abducted for a few seconds and then allowed to snap back (Rosselimo's sign) or a pin may be pricked onto the dorsum of the big toe. Finally you may have to use the patient's own thumb nail! All or any of these stimuli may provoke an extensor plantar response when it is present. If the big toe is immobile from joint disease or a lower motor neurone lesion, no movement can be expected. Fanning of the other toes and a contraction of the medial hamstring which can be palpated while scraping the foot may enable the clinician to estimate whether an extensor response would have occurred. A very easily detectable Babinski sign which appears to be present at rest is said to be likely to be due to multiple sclerosis. Likewise, bilateral extensor responses when symptoms are unilateral is suggestive of this diagnosis. In many indivi-

duals the toe fails to make a clear-cut movement in any direction.

The combination of absent ankle jerks and extensor plantar responses, much beloved by examiners, may be seen when a peripheral neuropathy occurs in a patient with an upper motor neurone lesion, e.g. a diabetic subject with cerebrovascular disease, or in AIDS. It can also be seen in tabes dorsalis, subacute combined degeneration of the cord, Friedreich's ataxia and with lesions of the conus medullaris, when cord and cauda equina are damaged together at the T12–L1 spinal level. The not uncommon coincidence of cervical and lumbar spondylosis is in practice one of the most usual causes.

The bulbocavernosus reflex (S3–5) is tested by palpating for contraction at the base of the penis whilst squeezing the glans, and the anal reflex (S4,5) consists of puckering of the skin as the anal sphincter contracts in response to pinprick or scratch of the perianal skin. The contraction of the external sphincter during this response can also be palpated by a gloved finger during the routine rectal examination. Both these reflexes are useful for testing patients with impotence or impaired sphincter function.

Tapping over nerves may produce tingling at sites of regeneration or compression (Tinel's sign) or twitching of muscles in hypocalcaemia. Chvostek's sign refers to such movements in the facial muscles on percussion over the facial nerve in the parotid bed in front of the ear.

Muscle power

The testing of individual muscles is shown in Figures 1.13–1.42. The required movement should be demonstrated to the patient and the correct position is crucial. In order to assess the power of muscles around the shoulder or hip, it is important that the patient's body is well supported and stable, either lying or seated. If the scapula is not held against the chest wall by the serratus, rhomboids and trapezius, for example, it may be necessary for the examiner to use a hand to help fix it by external pressure so that muscles like the deltoid may be tested

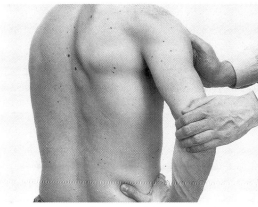

Figure 1.13 Backward rotation of the elbow in this position tests the rhomboids (C5–6).

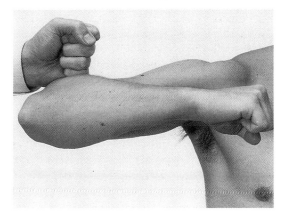

Figure 1.16 Abduction of the flexed elbow to the horizontal depends on the deltoid (C5).

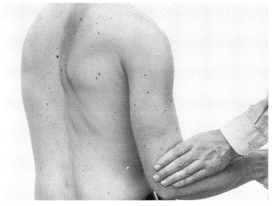

Figure 1.14 Abduction of the shoulder over the first few degrees is carried out by the supraspinatus (C5–6).

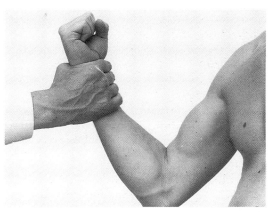

Figure 1.17 Flexion of the elbow tests the biceps (C5) when the forearm is supinated.

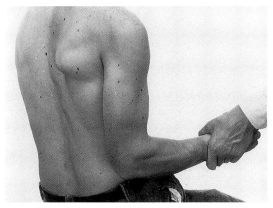

Figure 1.15 The examiner is attempting to roll the patient's arm across his chest. This movement is resisted by the infraspinatus (C5–6).

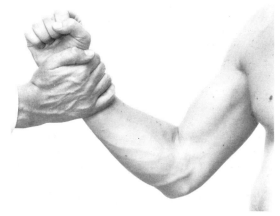

Figure 1.18 Flexion of the elbow with the forearm mid-pronated tests the brachioradialis (C6) supplied by the radial nerve.

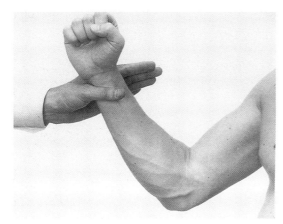

Figure 1.19 Extension of the elbow tests the triceps supplied by the radial nerve (C7).

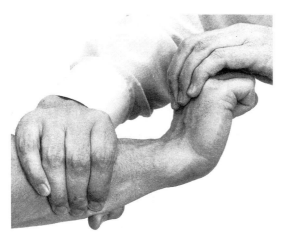

Figure 1.20 Resisted extension of the wrist tests radial (C7) supplied forearm extensor muscles.

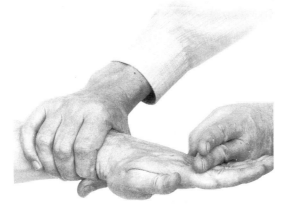

Figure 1.21 Extension of the fingers depends on radial nerve function (C7–8).

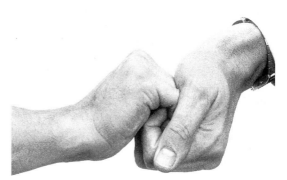

Figure 1.22 If median-supplied (C8) finger flexors are intact the curled fingers cannot be prized open by the examiner.

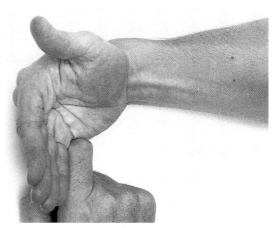

Figure 1.23 Flexion of the wrist on the ulnar side tests the ulnar supplied flexor carpi ulnaris.

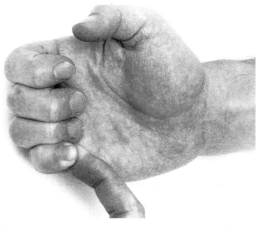

Figure 1.24 The ability to curl the tip of the little finger depends on an intact ulnar supply to the flexor digitorum profundus.

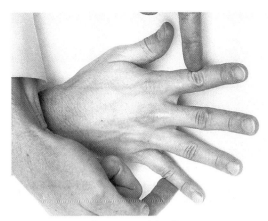

Figure 1.25 Forceful spread of the fingers against resistance tests the ulnar (T1) supplied intrinsic small hand muscles.

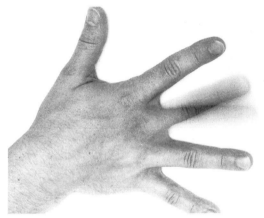

Figure 1.26 Rapid side-to-side movements of the middle finger can only be carried out if ulnar (T1) supplied interossei are normal.

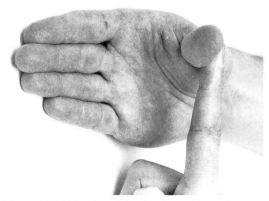

Figure 1.27 Abduction of the thumb at right angle to the palm is the best way to test the median (T1)-supplied abductor pollicis brevis, which is commonly weak in the carpal tunnel syndrome.

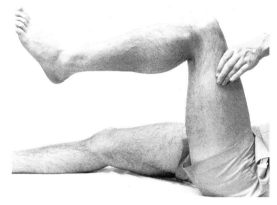

Figure 1.28 Flexion at the hip with the knee bent tests L2–3, supplying the iliopsoas.

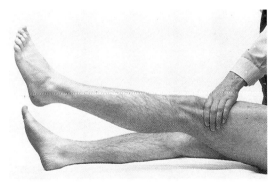

Figure 1.29 Elevation of the stiffened leg also tests hip flexion (L2–4) which is weak early on in an upper motor neurone lesion affecting the leg.

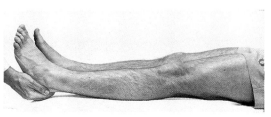

Figure 1.30 The patient is resisting the examiners attempt to lift the stiffened leg off the bed. This tests extension at the hip (L5–S1, sciatic nerve) which is relatively spared in upper motor neurone lesions.

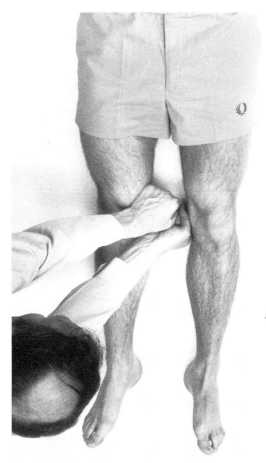

Figure 1.31 The examiner is attempting to overcome adduction at the hip (obdurator nerve, L3–4).

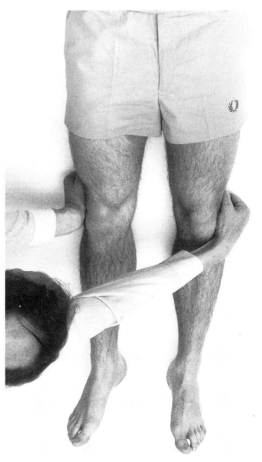

Figure 1.32 The examiner is resisting attempts to abduct at the hips (L5–S1).

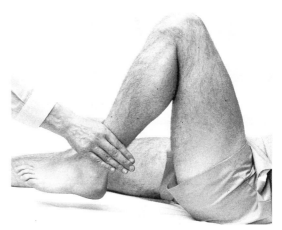

Figure 1.33 Extension of the knee by the quadriceps (femoral nerve L3–4).

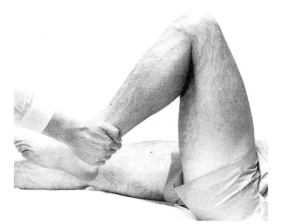

Figure 1.34 Flexion of the knee by the hamstrings (sciatic nerve L5–S1).

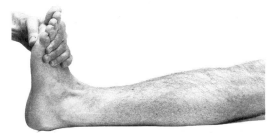

Figure 1.35 Dorsiflexion of the foot tests tibialis anterior supplied by the common peroneal nerve (L4–5). Weakness is seen early in upper motor neurone lesions affecting the leg.

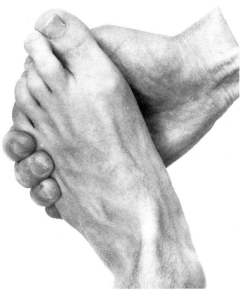

Figure 1.36 Resisted eversion of the foot tests the peronei supplied by the common peroneal nerve (L5–S1).

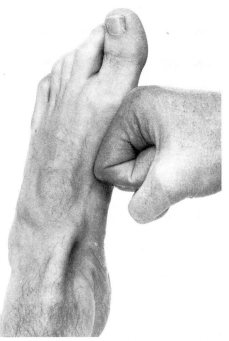

Figure 1.37 Forceful inversion of the foot is carried out by the tibialis anterior and posterior (L4).

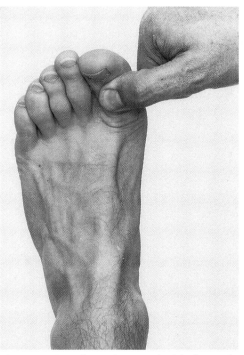

Figure 1.38 Dorsiflexion (extension) of the big toe by extensor hallucis longus is a good test of L5 innervated muscles.

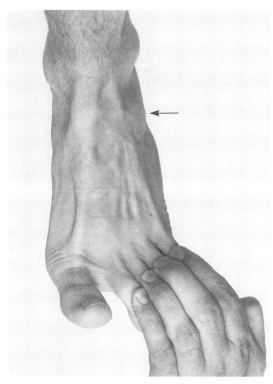

Figure 1.39 Dorsiflexion of the toes tests muscles supplied by the common peroneal nerve, including the extensor digitorum brevis (L5–S1) arrowed.

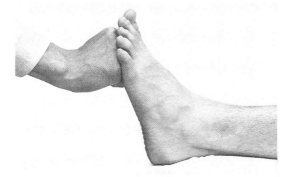

Figure 1.40 Plantar flexion of the foot is so strong that standing on tip toe is required to test it fully [posterior tibial nerve (S1)].

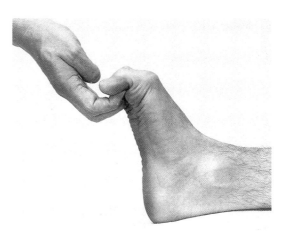

Figure 1.41 Long toe flexors are supplied by the posterior tibial nerve (S1).

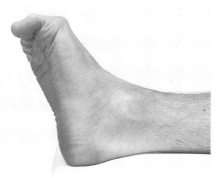

Figure 1.42 The ability to make a cup of the sole of the foot depends on intrinsic foot muscles such as abductor and flexor hallucis supplied by the posterior tibial nerve (S2).

properly. The loss of fixation seen for example in facioscapular muscular dystrophy leads to a striking physical sign when the patient holds his arms horizontally out to his sides. In this fully abducted position the tips of the scapulae

ride up and peep at the examiner over the top of the clavicles. In such a patient the true strength of muscles like the deltoid can be difficult to judge.

In all of the illustrations, the examiner's hand is resisting the movement whose power is being tested. In some cases, the second hand is needed to steady the patient's limb.

Recognizing full power is a matter of experience, and allowance has to be made in the young, the elderly and the ill. Pain may limit power around a diseased joint. Some muscles are normally so strong that they can resist the full power of the examiner using all his strength. For example, knee extension by the quadriceps and plantar flexion at the ankle by calf muscles cannot be tested fully on the bed. Rising from a deep squat or climbing stairs is a better test of the quadriceps, and standing on the toes of each foot is the best way to reveal early weakness of calf muscles. Standing on both heels can also reveal a partial foot drop. On the other hand, some muscles are easily overcome and one has to learn what to expect. Neck flexion is a good example of this and is overcome quite easily in all normal subjects. If it can be overcome with a single finger on the forehead, however, it is clearly pathologically weak.

In the case of limb muscles the degree of shortening of the muscle makes a significant difference to the examiner's ability to overcome its contraction. For example, if the triceps is tested with the elbow nearly straight, it is very difficult to overcome. If the patient is instructed to flex the elbow fully, then even a normal triceps can be resisted by gentle restraint. The quadriceps is also too powerful to test in the nearly straight kneed position advocated by some. It is best to test muscles at the same position in all cases so as to build up a personal 'feel' for strength in the normal situation. In most cases this will involve testing the movement in its midpoint with joints at 90° in the case of the shoulder, elbow, hip and knee. The routine position for testing distal muscles is shown in the figures. The greater weakness of muscles when their belly is at its longest can be turned to the examiner's advantage. For example, a slightly weak tibialis anterior may still be able to resist attempts to depress the fully dorsiflexed ankle, but its ability to begin that movement from a starting point of full plantar flexion may reveal its loss of power. When pain limits movement or the patient's nervous state impairs co-operation, one has to lower one's sights as far as checking power is concerned. Some normal activities are proof of normal power; getting out of bed or up from a chair, for example. Any brief movement of full power when testing implies that there is no fixed weakness and this can often be judged, for example before the patient's pain prevents continued movement.

Some movements involve more than one muscle. The usual way to test hip extension (Figure 1.31) in fact tests gluteus maximus and hamstrings together. If it is necessary to isolate the gluteus the patient should be turned prone and hip extension tested with the knee flexed to 90° degrees. (This manoeuvre tends to cause cramp even in normals.)

When testing elevation of one leg off the bed, it is helpful to have a hand under the other lower leg. This can then detect that the patient is really trying to lift the one leg since the movement is then accompanied by extension of the other limb. Lack of such counter-extension implies lack of co-operation and raises doubts over any weakness. This 'trick' is very useful when dealing with unilateral weakness. It is obviously less helpful when there is bilateral weakness, though even here if the strength of hip extensors acting as prime movers is much less than when elevating the contralateral leg, there is again evidence of incomplete effort.

It is convenient to record muscle power using the Medical Research Council scale: 0 = not even a flicker of movement; 1 = a visible flicker of contraction but no movement; 2 = a movement but not against gravity; 3 = a movement against gravity; 4 = a movement against resistance; and 5 = normal power. This scale was designed to follow recovery after nerve injury and is insensitive to degrees of weakness against resistance commonly encountered in clinical practice. Some physicians refer to 4.75, 4.5 and 4.25 or to 4+++, 4++, 4+ to refer to mild, moderate and severe weakness, though still all against resistance.

When testing patients with long-standing focal weakness, for example after a peripheral nerve lesion, one should be aware of 'trick movements'. Patients subconsciously 'learn' to simulate the action of a paralysed muscle by the use of others. These can be detected by attention to detail and palpation of muscle bellies while testing.

Truncal muscles

The patient should be asked to attempt to sit up from the lying position. This calls for contraction of the muscles of the anterior abdominal wall which should be observed and palpated. If the umbilicus shifts upwards this suggests that the lower muscles are weaker than the upper, as with a lesion at about T10. The thoracic cage should be observed during respiration if a muscle disorder or thoracic cord lesion is suspected. A lesion at T6, say, may paralyse lower intercostal muscles which will be indrawn passively during respiration. Damage to the phrenic nerves may be obvious as paradoxical movement of the abdominal wall during respiration due to loss of descent of the diaphragm during inspiration. The vital capacity in these circumstances is much different when recorded supine and seated.

Upper motor neurone weakness

If an upper motor neurone disturbance is suspected, then increases in tone and reflexes can be expected and a particular pattern of weakness is found.

In the upper limb shoulder abduction, elbow extension, wrist and finger extension and finger separation are weaker than their antagonists. Thus patients might show a slight weakness of the deltoid, triceps and of finger extension with normal adduction of the shoulder, biceps and grip. Voluntary movements are lost before automatic ones, so the arm paralysed by an acute stroke may still move during a yawn, for example.

With cortical lesions there may be striking loss of the ability to make discrete movements, for example of a single digit. If the patient is asked to hold both arms fully extended at shoulder level in front of him, with his palms upwards, the upper motor neurone weakness may be revealed by a tendency to pronation of the forearm on the affected side when he closes his eyes. The arm may also drift but this also happens with joint position sense loss, so this is not specific. The ability to carry out rapid movements of the fingers, for example when pretending to play the piano, is impaired with cortical lesions particularly.

In the leg, the weaker movement at each main joint is of hip flexion, knee flexion, dorsiflexion and eversion of the foot. A patient may be unable to lift the leg off the bed and have a foot drop at a time when hip extension and

quadriceps are normal and he can stand on 'tiptoe'. As he walks the leg is swung out in an arc and the inturned dropped foot trails on the ground. The hip is hitched up to aid clearance of the ground given the weakness of lift in the knee and foot.

Clearly, with an acute devastating stroke all movement may be lost in the limb. In the first few days after such a stroke the limb may be flaccid and show no increase in reflexes. The extensor plantar response elicited by scraping the lateral margin of the sole of the foot with an orange stick may be the only proof of the upper motor neurone lesion responsible. Bilateral movements like those of the larynx, pharynx, thorax and abdomen are little affected. Acute spinal cord damage as after trauma may also fail to show the classical signs of upper motor neurone lesion to begin with due to a condition called spinal shock, which causes flaccidity and arreflexia below the lesion for some days.

The posture of the long-established hemiplegic limbs, the flexed arm held to the side, and the extended leg swung in an arc to limit the dragging of the inverted toes on the ground, is a good aide-memoire for the distribution of weakness found at an early stage when examining the patient on the couch. Other patterns of weakness that are also revealing are the symmetrical proximal distribution of weakness in myopathies and the peripheral, i.e. distal, weakness in peripheral neuropathy. Knowledge of nerve root and peripheral nerve territories is needed to distinguish weakness of restricted distribution due to isolated lower motor neurone problems. There is no shame attached to 'looking them up'.

Further reading

MAYO CLINIC AND MAYO FOUNDATION (1991) *Clinical Examinations in Neurology*, 6th edn. W.B. Mosby Year Book, St Louis.
MEDICAL RESEARCH COUNCIL (1990) *Aids to the Examination of the Peripheral Nervous System*. Baillière Tindall, London.

Extrapyramidal system

The basal ganglia are involved in motor control, and perhaps in motor programming. Their damage affects the tone of muscles, the rapidity of muscle contraction and postural control. The initiation of walking and its alternating pattern of limb movement require shifts of the centre of gravity forward and from side to side. Also, any sudden displacement needs corrective adjustments of body posture to prevent falls. These functions are therefore likely to be affected by basal ganglia disorders. In addition, involuntary movements of various sorts are common.

The archetypal basal ganglia disorder is Parkinson's disease, which shows many of these phenomena. The patient's gait is characteristic, with a flexed posture, lack of arm swing and reduced stride. The arm is semiflexed at the elbow. The patient's feet appear glued to the floor, especially when passing through a doorway. To start walking the parkinsonian patient shuffles his feet with small stuttering steps. Assistance in propelling the body forward and rocking the pelvis from side to side helps, as do visual clues, for example well-spaced lines on the floor. The face becomes impassive and the body increasingly flexed. They may lie in bed with their head off the pillow. Movements occur 'en bloc' like those of a wooden doll. The voice becomes quiet, monotonous and when severely affected, mumbling and incoherent. Eating and swallowing may become slow and difficult, leading to dribbling.

Both the trunk and limbs show muscular rigidity. Throughout the range of passive flexion and extension of the wrist or elbow, a stiffness is felt like bending a piece of lead pipe. This contrasts with the asymmetrical catch of increased tone in biceps rather than triceps in spasticity due to unchecked spinal reflex activity with upper motor neurone lesions. Axial muscles also show rigidity, detectable in the neck if it is passively flexed and extended. Movements are slowed, and this is well seen in the patient's attempt to oppose each finger in turn on the tip of the thumb, or to rapidly tap the tip of the thumb with the tip of the index. The movements are small in range and get progressively smaller until the thumb is sliding over the other fingertips. This is usually called poverty of movement but economy is a better word for it since the task is correctly performed though with a greatly limited range. Handwriting gets smaller and smaller down the page of a letter. Tapping on the floor with either foot whilst sitting reveals comparable difficulties with the lower limb.

A repeated tap with a finger on the midforehead produces repeated blinking in the parkinsonian patient (glabellar tap sign), a response that habituates in the normal after only one or two trials. The examiner's hand must be held over the forehead from behind lest its movement elicits a blink to a visual threat. The basis of this glabellar tap sign is unknown. It contrasts with the diminished frequency of spontaneous blinking in this condition.

If the shoulders of the standing patient are alternately swung fore and aft by the examiner putting his hands on each shoulder, the lack of swing of the dependent arm can reveal unilateral parkinsonian rigidity at an early stage. The patient may have a mild scoliosis with unilateral parkinsonism. The slowness of movement produces spurious weakness. If the patient is not given time to contract a muscle it appears weak.

Tremor, defined as a rhythmical oscillation of a body part, is usual and affects distal parts of the limb, commonly beginning in one hand. The thumb and fingers show a regular oscillation at 4–6 Hz. This tremor is most marked when the limb is at rest, e.g. lying on the lap when seated or by the side when standing or walking. The tremor lessens with full relaxation and disappears in sleep. It is often asymmetrical. It gives to the increased tone of the limb a ratchet or cogwheel feel.

Tremor on maintenance of the outstretched posture of the arms and when holding a paper or cup and saucer is sometimes misdiagnosed as Parkinson's disease without other physical signs, when it is in fact due to benign essential tremor, an often familial condition. The legs are involved in only a minority, but there is often a nodding tremor of the head (titubation), and voice. The head may nod or rock from side to side. The tremor of the voice is revealed by cajoling the patient into singing a sustained 'Ahhh'. This 'essential' tremor tends to be improved by alcohol and may respond to propranolol or primidone. By contrast, the tremor of Parkinson's disease is as noted, a rest tremor, and is usually accompanied by rigidity, postural change, or slowing. It may affect the lips and tongue rather than the head. Rarely an isolated tremor causes difficulty in diagnosis for 1–2 years before the other parkinsonian features appear. A tremor of the legs like essential tremor may develop only on standing (orthostatic tremor). Isolated tremors of the voice, tongue, chin, face, writing, or trunk are probably also versions of essential tremor, as is that accompanying hereditary neuropathy.

A fine rapid tremor is detected in the outstretched fingers of normal subjects (physiological tremor). This becomes exaggerated by thyrotoxicosis and some drugs. Attention to the circumstances under which tremor is detected (Table 1.13) is the best prelude to deciding on its cause (Table 1.14). A sheet of paper placed on the outstretched fingers helps to reveal the frequency of fine tremors such as those of thyrotoxicosis.

Cerebellar disease (see below) causes a slower, irregular, and often more proximal tremor due to inco-ordination of movement. Though it may be seen on maintenance of a posture, it is most marked whilst carrying out a planned movement as in the finger–nose–finger test. Lesions of the cerebellar outflow (peduncles, etc.) as caused by multiple sclerosis, Wilson's disease, and tumours can cause a dramatic wing-beating tremor of the outstretched arm to which is added an intentional element on action.

Table 1.13 Types of tremor

	Rest	Posture	Action
Parkinson's disease*	+++	+	– –
Essential tremor	– –	+++	+
Cerebellar	– –	+	+++
Cerebellar peduncle	– –	+++	+++
Physiological Thyrotoxicosis Anxiety	– –	+	– –

* Rarely develops on action.

Table 1.14 Causes of tremor

Condition of limb	Cause
Rest	Parkinson's disease
Maintenance of unsupported posture, e.g. outstretched hands	Physiological Anxiety Thyrotoxicosis Essential tremor Drugs: Alcohol Lithium Sodium valproate Amphetamines Sympathomimetics
On movement, e.g. finger/ nose test	Cerebellar lesion
On posture and movement	Cerebellar peduncle lesion, e.g. multiple sclerosis

Table 1.15 Movement disorders

Nomenclature	Definition/description
Asterixis	Flap due to losses of postural tone
Athetosis	Wavering movements usually distal
Pseudo-athetosis	Same but due to position sense loss
Ballism	Flinging movements usually proximal
Chorea	Random jerky movements
Dystonia	Spasms and postural distortions
Myoclonus	Shock-like muscle twitch
Myokymia	Writhing bag of worms
Tremor	Rhythmical oscillation about a joint

Basal ganglia lesions cause other involuntary movements (Table 1.15).

Deposition of copper (Wilson's disease) causes a mixture of tremor and abnormal posturing (torsion spasms or dystonia) which often involve movements about the long axis of the limb producing internal rotation of the forearm and a similar twisting of the foot usually accompanied by persistent extension of the big toe. Dystonia may also be seen after hemiplegia due to head injury or stroke, and may also develop and become generalized in the condition dystonia musculorum deformans. Dystonic movements are prominent amongst the involuntary movements induced by L-dopa in patients with Parkinson's disease, usually after a few years' treatment. They are dose dependent.

Torticollis refers to rotation and tilting of the head, which can be tonic or spasmodic or both. Usually no pathology is discernible.

Paresis of the muscles in spasm produced by injections of botulinum toxin can control the condition.

Fleeting muscle contractions looking like mannerisms but flitting from one place to another are called choreic movements, and are seen in rheumatic chorea, in pregnancy and occasionally in those taking the contraceptive pill, or in systemic lupus erythematosus. Chorea with dementia characterizes the dominantly inherited Huntington's chorea, the gene for which has been located on chromosome 4. The movements may cause respiratory irregularity, explosive speech and an inability to protrude the tongue steadily ('darting tongue'). The hand grip may be interrupted by muscle contractions ('milk maid grip'). Choreiform movements occur randomly and are not predictable by the examiner. The differential diagnosis of chorea includes tics or habit spasms. These are predictable and one can look out for repetitions of movements in the eyebrow, face or neck, for example. The patient can prevent these briefly by an act of will but at the expense of a sense of mounting inner tension. In the Gilles de la Tourette syndrome involuntary expletives and sounds are added to motor tics. There is a link with obsessional–compulsive behaviour traits.

Athetosis refers to distal digital movements and is rare as an isolated movement disorder. It is more often seen combined with dystonic posturing or chorea. Pseudoathetosis refers to a similar wavering of outstretched fingers due to severe joint position sense loss and is commonly seen with dorsal root entry zone changes in multiple sclerosis. The term choreoathetosis should be avoided as a portmanteau word that fails to define the type of movement seen.

Hemiballismus consists of violent flinging movements of the limbs on one side due to a lesion near or in the subthalamic nucleus, commonly an infarct. The patients are often elderly and become exhausted. (The movements may be dampened by the use of tetrabenazine or by a stereotactic thalamotomy.)

Myoclonic jerks are sudden explosive contractions of muscles as though in response to electric shock stimulation of their motor nerves. They are seen in metabolic disorders (uraemia, for example), in epilepsy sometimes triggered by photic stimulation, and in some hereditary conditions, as well as with degenerations of the dentate nucleus and olivary complex. Some infective conditions (subacute sclerosing panencephalitis, Creutzfeld–Jakob disease) are characterized by regular myoclonus. Rarely, myoclonus arises from a spinal cord lesion. Single jerks of the legs at the point of dropping off to sleep are described by many normal people and are considered physiological.

Flickering in the face may be of different types. A fine but irritating flicker in the eyelid is a common, almost physiological event related to fatigue. Widespread continuous undulating or rippling contraction of one side of the face (myokymia) can be seen with brain-stem lesions like multiple sclerosis. A lesion of the facial nerve, for example in the cerebellopontine angle or after a Bell's palsy, may cause a coarser more intermittent twitching of the face (hemifacial spasm) in which tonic contraction of the face causes the affected cheek to be drawn up. There is usually mild weakness as well. Rhythmic twitching of one corner of the mouth or of the eyes may be seen with focal epileptic activity. An EEG will reveal this cause of facial movement as 'epilepsia partialis continuans'. Involuntary closure of the eyelids (blepharospasm) is probably a focal kind of dystonia. Partial section of the facial nerve or injections of botulinum toxin may be needed to control it. Grimacing of the face may be combined with writhing movements of the tongue (orofacial dyskinesia) and is commonly due to phenothiazine medication. Some patients make a stereotyped movement of the face out of habit (a tic).

Dystonia

Agonists and antagonists both contract, causing muscle spasms that distort the limb into characteristic postures. The head may be tilted, rotated or retracted (torticollis or retrocollis) and the back rotated or tilted (tortipelvis), the arm internally rotated with extended fingers and the leg extended with an inverted foot whose big toe is extended. Postures such as these may be maintained or appear briefly during spasms which are often triggered by movement.

The commonest cause of dystonia encountered in everyday practice is the use of L-dopa in the treatment of Parkinson's disease. The dystonic spasms appear as a dose-dependent side-effect. When a patient with Parkinson's disease on treatment with L-dopa complains of a deterioration in walking, it is important to distinguish between a progression of their disease and the development of dystonic posturing of the leg and foot. The extended big toe or clawing of the little toes due to dystonia will usually have been noted by the patient or can be seen while watching the patient walk. Dystonia can also result from phenothiazines.

Primary or idiopathic dystonia musculorum deformans is inherited as an autosomal dominant disorder with incomplete penetrance and is more common in Ashkenazi Jews. Onset is in childhood, usually with posturing of the foot when walking. The condition is progressive, at least in the early years, and comes to affect all four limbs and axial structures.

Rarer causes of dystonia include copper deposition (Wilson's disease) in which rigidity and tremor are accompanied by dysarthria and impaired intelligence. The condition presents before the age of 20 and is diagnosed by slit lamp examination for a Kayser–Fleischer corneal stain which causes a brown ring around the outer rim, and assay of blood caeruloplasmin levels. It has been associated with chromosome 13. Gangliosidoses, Hallervorden–Spatz disease, Leigh's disease, and neuroacanthocytosis can be sporadic or hereditary causes of chorea, vocal tics, and oromandibular dystonia which can cause self-mutilation. Infarcts or tumours in the basal ganglia are also rare causes. Focal lesions are most likely to be relevant in adults whose dystonia usually begins in and stays confined to an upper limb. Involuntary eye closure (blepharospasm) may cause disability by impairing vision. It begins with excessive blinking in response to bright light and stress. It may be momentarily relieved by yawning. It can be thought of as a forme fruste of generalized dystonia, as can task specific dystonias. The commonest of these affects writing: a dystonic posture of the arm only developing during the act of writing. A childhood dystonia showing marked fluctuation throughout the day is important to recognize as it is dramatically responsive to small doses of L-dopa.

Further reading

MARSDEN, C.D. AND FAHN, S. (1994) *Movement Disorders 3*. Butterworth-Heinemann, London.

HARDING, A.E. (1994) *Genetics in Neurology*. Baillière Tindall, London.

Cerebellar function

It is important to realize that the tests in everyday clinical use are not specific. Thus impairment due to sensory loss can mimic the effect of disease of the cerebellum or its connections. The distinction depends on observing whether the patient's problems are the same with eyes open or closed (cerebellar deficit) or much improved by visual attention (joint position sense loss). Patients with sensory rather than cerebellar ataxia also show odd posturing of the outstretched hands and fingers with closed eyes (pseudo-athetosis), and of course have sensory loss when tested. If the limbs are very weak, many of the cerebellar tests cannot be interpreted with any safety.

Abnormalities of cerebellar hemispheres produce ipsilateral disturbance of limb co-ordination. This is best tested by the ability to make a smooth and accurate tracking movement with an outstretched finger from a distant target such as the examiner's upheld finger, to the patient's nose: the finger–nose–finger test. The patient must not be allowed to tuck his elbow into his side to steady the movement, and the finger target must be sufficiently far away to force the patient to reach out fully. If the patient cannot see, the task is restricted to asking him to touch the tip of his nose with the tip of his index finger, the examiner determining the start position by holding the patient's arm outstretched. Clearly the test cannot be carried out if the arm is too weak to hold itself up against gravity. Oscillation of the limb, especially on reaching either target, is a sign of cerebellar malfunction. If the limb is severely ataxic the opposition of the finger to the nose should be omitted for fear the patient damages his eye. It is enough to have the patient reach out for the examiner's hand in this situation.

It is also revealing to ask the patient to tap on the back of one hand with the palmar aspect of the fingers of the other. This can normally be done rhythmically and rapidly, though there is usually a little asymmetry, the non-dominant hand being a little less fluent. Some difficulty with this tapping task is seen in Parkinson's disease, but in a limb affected by cerebellar problems the hand movement is chaotic (dysdiadochokinesis), and the elbow moves unnecessarily. The poor rhythm can be seen and heard. Similarly, the patient can be asked to rotate the forearm rapidly to and fro as though rattling a doorknob. This movement is slowed and lacks rhythm in the presence of a cerebellar hemisphere lesion. Finally, if the arms are held extended at the shoulder level and tapped downwards by the examiner, the affected side may be displaced by a greater amount. The patient's drawing of a spiral may also reveal irregularities of co-ordination and his writing is untidy and large.

In the lower limbs the ability to place one heel accurately on the other knee and then run it down the anterior ridge of the tibia is tested: the heel-knee-shin test. When defective, the heel waves from side to side and falls off the tibial edge. The movement of lowering the heel onto the knee may also be visibly 'wobbly'. Patients should be allowed to have more than one attempt at the task as it requires a little practice. Don't be content with a rapid movement of the externally rotated foot down the side of the calf. Regular tapping of the floor with either foot when sitting may also reveal irregularity. Again, joint position sense loss impairs these lower limb tests of co-ordination but in that case visual attention corrects the errors, which in the case of cerebellar disease remain the same with eyes open or closed.

With disease of the cerebellar connections in the brain stem, a vertical nodding tremor of the head may be seen (titubation), but this is also seen in benign essential tremor in which there is no known cerebellar pathology. The tremor seen with lesions of the cerebellar ped-

uncle and brain-stem connections shows a combination of tremor on maintenance of outstretched hands, and on the finger–nose–finger test. It tends to have a to-and-fro movement at the shoulder, and a side to side movement at the wrist, as if the patient were polishing the top of a table. It is seen in multiple sclerosis, Wilson's disease, brain-stem infarction, and with the toxicity of phenytoin and alcohol.

Midline cerebellar lesions cause midline ataxia, i.e. of stance and gait, rather than striking limb ataxia. The ability to stand with feet close together and walk both normally and heel-to-toe as on a tightrope is tested. Cerebellar deficit is revealed by the need to widen the base and a tendency to stagger or totter from side to side. Some unsteadiness on heel-toe walking can occur if the patient is tense and is to be expected in the elderly. Turning may be especially revealing. Again a similar imbalance is produced by position sense loss but the effect of eye closure is again helpful. If the ability to stand still with feet together is lost with eye closure (Romberg's sign positive), the deficit is due to joint position sense loss. If imbalance is present whether or not the eyes are open, cerebellar function is faulty. Before getting the patient to carry out the Romberg test, ask yourself whether you will be able to stop them falling if it is dramatically positive! If they are too big and heavy, seek assistance. A small degree of sway with eyes closed is normal, and anxious patients show exaggerated movement and immediately open their eyes and grip hold of the examiner. The test can therefore be difficult to assess.

The much described veering to one side with a unilateral cerebellar hemisphere tumour is rarely seen, and certainly its absence is of little import. Sometimes there is some spasm of neck muscles on the side of a cerebellar mass lesion which may cause head tilt (Cairns' sign). The differential diagnosis of head tilt also includes vertical diplopia, for example due to a fourth nerve palsy, a painful disorder of the cervical spine and the involuntary movement disease torticollis. Cerebellar disease also disturbs the co-ordination of bulbar muscles, causing slurring dysarthria, and of eye movements. As the eyes return to the central position from a lateral deviation, the fixation point is overshot and the eye oscillates briefly before stabilizing on the new target. Nystagmus to the side may also be seen.

Imbalance of stance and gait with less obvious limb ataxia usually proves to be due to a midline cerebellar mass or to diffuse cerebellar lesions. Unilateral limb ataxia indicative of an ipsilateral cerebellar lesion is usually due to a focal lesion. The differential diagnosis of ataxia starts with separating those due to loss of joint position sense from those with cerebellar signs. In the latter context one has to consider strokes, tumours, congenital abnormalities like the Arnold–Chiari malformation with cerebellar tonsillar descent through the foramen magnum, and abscesses (Table 1.16). Wernicke's encephalopathy, Creutzfeld–Jakob disease, paraneoplastic

syndromes and hereditary conditions like Friedreich's ataxia are rarer causes. The sudden development of a cerebellar syndrome should suggest a stroke; the rapid progression of cerebellar signs on the other hand is suspicious of Creutzfeld–Jakob disease and a paraneoplastic syndrome. (Rarely, in bronchial carcinoma an equally disabling ataxia may develop due to sensory loss, because of inflammatory change in dorsal root ganglia.)

Further reading

LECHTENBERG, R. (ed.) (1993) *The Handbook of Cerebellar Disease*. Marcel Dekker, New York.

Sensation

The complaint of numbness may or may not refer to loss of sensation. Some patients use 'numb' to refer to an aching discomfort, weakness, clumsiness, inco-ordination or strangeness, and they must be interrogated until it is as clear as possible whether sensory change is being described. Disturbances of small fibre function in peripheral nerves or of spinothalamic tracts may give rise to the complaints of pain, burning, coldness or the feeling of running cold water on the skin. Disturbances of sensation carried by large fibres and in the posterior columns of the spinal cord particularly give rise to complaints of numbness, pins and needles, walking on cotton wool, deadness and tight bands around the extremities or trunk. High-level lesions, for example in the parietal cortex, may give rise to a feeling that the limb does not belong to the patient or has a will of its own, appearing in positions not realized by the patient until his attention is drawn to it.

The sensory examination is often difficult, time consuming, and frustrating, though also revealing. If a screening examination is all that is required (to detect any unsuspected abnormality), it may be enough to test symmetrical appreciation of the light touch of a fingertip and a pin on all four limbs, plus awareness of movements of the big toe and tip of an index finger on either side. Joint

Table 1.16 Causes of cerebellar impairment

Diagnosis	Clues
Ataxia telangiectasia	Children, telangiectasia eyes, skin
Olivopontocerebellar degeneration	Parkinsonism + cerebellar deficit + sphincter impairment + dementia
Cerebellar degeneration	± dementia, slow evolution
Alcohol abuse	± neuropathy, liver disease
Hypothyroidism	Slow relaxing tendon jerks
Drugs	Phenytoin, mercury, 5 flucytosine, methotrexate + radiotherapy
Myoclonic epilepsy	Seizures, myoclonus + cerebellar signs
Underlying malignancy	Bronchus, ovary especially
Infectious mononucleosis	Febrile illness, lymphadenopathy
Heat stroke	Circumstances
Coeliac disease	Associated neuropathy, malabsorption
Tumour	Headache, vomiting, papilloedema
Legionella pneumonia	Atypical pneumonia, confusion, increased creatine kinase activity
Arnold–Chiari malformation (foramen magnum)	Downbeat nystagmus, short neck
Friedreich's ataxia	Onset in second decade, scoliosis, loss ankle jerks, extensor plantars, pes cavus, cardiomyopathy, impaired joint position sense chromosome 9.

position sense should always be tested, since its loss may be silent, i.e. unaccompanied by suggestive symptoms. If a hemisphere lesion is suspected even when there are no sensory symptoms, it is still worth testing for inattention. Both sides are touched and the patient with his eyes closed is asked to report whether he feels the stimulus on either or both sides. Patients with parietal lobe lesions may have intact sensation (tested one side at a time) but 'miss' on the contralateral limbs when given simultaneous stimuli.

When more detailed testing is needed all modalities should be explored. Such an examination is trying for both examiner and patient, and to give the patient a rest it may be wise to interrupt it, perhaps while listening to the heart or palpating the abdomen. Touch can be assessed by a fingertip, which has the advantage that the examiner gets some feedback on how firm a touch was delivered, or with cotton wool when greater sensitivity is required. The touch of a fine wisp of wool may be appreciated on the face, as is used for testing corneal sensation and the corneal reflex, but for the limbs a bulkier piece of cotton wool is needed. It should be dabbed on to the skin, not run along it or stroked as the latter may involve the alternate sensation of tickle allied to pain. All four limbs should be tested as a routine. If a spinal cord lesion is suspected, the trunk also should be tested for a level below which touch is impaired. If a root or peripheral nerve lesion seems likely, the territory of the appropriate nerve or root and its neighbours and its contralateral partner should be compared. Sensation should be assessed, starting in the abnormal area and working towards the normal. The area of paraesthesiae usually exceeds the area of objective change and the area of loss of light touch sensation is normally greater than the area of pinprick loss. Hard skin over the soles of the feet makes them insensitive to cotton wool.

To test pain sensation, the sting of a pinprick is used. A different pin should be used for each patient in case blood is drawn, although this should not happen. It may be revealing to ask the patient to say whether the sharp or blunt end of the pin is in use. Some areas are naturally more sensitive to the pin, such as the root of the neck, nipples, the inner arms and groins. The pulp of the finger is less sensitive than the tip and nail bed, which are the preferred areas to test on the hands. Again all four limbs should be tested. Any abnormality in the lower limbs or other clue to spinal cord disease then requires the search for a 'level' on the trunk. Pinprick testing produces a sharper level than with other modalities, and is the best choice for mapping areas of sensory loss.

Joint position sense is normally tested in the fingertips and toes. The tip of the digit is held between the examiner's thumb and index. The patient is shown how an upward and downward movement will be made and how he will be asked to report the direction once his eyes are closed. Small movements should be made initially. Some patients report up and down alternately, regardless of the examiner's choice. Before concluding that this is evidence of loss of appreciation of joint movement, one should check that the patient can score correctly when allowed to watch the movement. Then go back to testing with the patient's eyes closed. Some patients will not close their eyes and an assistant has to put a hand over their eyes or the patient must be asked to hold a newspaper up in front of his face whilst joint position sense in the toes is being tested. Normal subjects can detect small displacements of about 2 mm in the tips of the fingers, and 5 mm in the tip of the big toe.

If a patient has genuine difficulty with small movements of terminal phalanges, large movements or movements of more proximal joints should be tested. The ability to shoot accurately at one's big toe with an index finger despite the foot being repositioned by the examiner tests position sense at more proximal joints. Joint position sense may be impaired in some digits and not others, for example in cervical root lesions, so in this context it may be worth testing more than one finger.

Vibration sense can be tested with a tuning fork. Its base should be pressed on the back of the terminal phalanx of the index and tip of hallux and the patient asked if he can feel a vibration. If the fork is 'twanged' too hard by the examiner before placing it on the patient, there may be confusion between hearing and feeling, and this must be avoided. If the fork cannot be felt on the toe it should be placed on the medial malleolus, tibial tuberosity, anterior iliac crest, rib margin, sternum or clavicles and up the vertebral column in the search for a level. Old people cannot feel vibration in the foot and sometimes at the ankle so loss needs to be interpreted with caution. A 128 Hz fork must be used, not the high-pitched fork used to test hearing (512 Hz). Loss may be a very sensitive indicator of spinal cord compression as in cervical myelopathy from spondylosis, or in a peripheral neuropathy such as that associated with diabetes. Root lesions can cause effects on vibration sense in different fingers.

Two-point threshold changes are especially useful in detecting problems restricted to the digits supplied by one peripheral nerve. Again, the test should be demonstrated to the patient with his eyes open before assessing the minimum separation he can accurately detect with eyes closed. In the pulp of the fingers a separation of 3–4 mm is normal, on the sole of the foot 3–4 cm. If the patient persistently reports feeling both blunt ends of the two-point discriminator when only one is applied, they should be advised to say 'one' when in doubt, and the test restarted, including some wide separations about which there is no doubt before 'homing' in on the threshold. Co-operation can also be checked, for example when testing the sole of the foot, by rocking the discriminator from one point onto the other to be sure the patient is reporting accurately.

Temperature testing is required only if a lesion of the spinothalamic pathway or small fibre neuropathy is suspected. A crude check can be made using the metal of the tuning fork or the head of the tendon hammer which feel cold, but if more detail is required special metal tubes filled with either warm or cold water are used to map areas of impaired recognition.

Modern equipment is now becoming available to provide quantitative data on thresholds, for example to vibration and temperature.

Patients with hysterical sensory loss are difficult to assess, but as with weakness of nonorganic origin, inconsistency is marked. Also, the patches of numbness may not match any known anatomical boundaries. A useful feature is the exact midline boundary that they often report which is usually not seen with organic hemianaesthesia. Vibration sense may be declared absent on one side of the midline when the fork is applied to either side of the sternum or frontal bone even though the vibration will of course cross the midline to the 'good side'. Patients may also produce a dramatic NO each and every time they are touched when asked to report if they feel a stimulus with their eyes closed! Such patients can easily be persuaded that an area is numb and later that it is not.

Patients with cortical lesions have extra difficulties that help locate their source of sensory disturbance. They have difficulty localizing tactile stimuli, cannot 'read' a number drawn on the tip of the thumb or on the palm (graphasthaesia) and despite intact crude sensation cannot identify an object such as a coin placed in the hand with their eyes closed. If the hand is paralysed the examiner must move the coin about in the subject's hand to provide the exploratory part of the normal strategy in identifying objects (stereognosis). The ability to detect, discriminate and identify different textures may also be lost, the seamstress being no longer able to rummage in her work basket and pick out a piece of satin or velvet, without looking at what she has in her hand. A unilateral disturbance of light touch, joint position sense and localization is found contralateral to the affected parietal lobe (Figure 1.43). The phenomenon of inattention may be detected (see above). Cerebral lesions may cause patchy sensory loss in the face or in individual digits. Extension of sensory loss to the trunk suggests a deeper lesion, for example in the thalamus.

Lesions of descending inhibitory pathways near or in the thalamus may lead to thalamic pain felt on the opposite side of the body. The threshold to pain may be elevated, but when reached the stimulus provokes a much nastier, more distressing, longer lasting and more diffuse pain than does a pinprick on the normal side. In the brain stem spinothalamic loss may affect one side of the face and the opposite limbs (Figure 1.44).

Lesions in the spinal cord may also affect the spinothalamic tract and spare the posterior

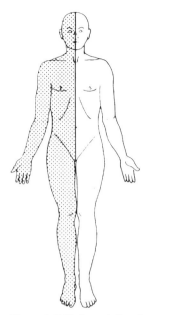

Figure 1.43 Unilateral disturbance affecting light touch, joint position sense and localization owing to a thalamic lesion.

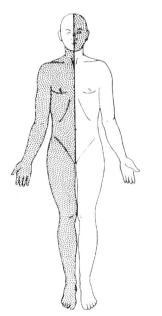

Figure 1.44 Crossed sensory loss with impaired pain and temperature sensation on one side of the face and the opposite side of the body is indicative of an intrinsic brain-stem lesion.

columns (Figure 1.45), e.g. in syringomyelia (Figure 1.46). This produces dissociated sensory loss affecting pain and temperature rather than joint position sense (Figure 1.47). With a unilateral cord lesion (Figure 1.48) there may be impairment of power (upper motor neurone) and joint position and two-point discrimination on one side and loss of pain and temperature appreciation on the other (Brown–Sequard syndrome) (Figure 1.49). The usual effect of a cord lesion is, however, a sensory 'level' below which all modalities are impaired (Figure 1.50) e.g. T4 at the nipple, T8 at the rib cage, and T10 at the umbilicus. The boundary may be indistinct, however, and may be one or two dermatomes lower than the responsible spinal pathology. In the days before sophisticated neuroradiology, laminectomies for spinal cord tumour were often carried out one or two vertebrae too low when the diagnosis depended on the

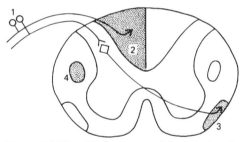

Figure 1.45 Simplified anatomy of the spinal cord. 1 = Dorsal root ganglion cells. 2 = Dorsal column. 3 Spinothalamic tract. 4 = Corticospinal tract.

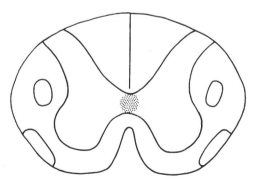

Figure 1.46 Expansion of the central canal (hydromyelia, syringomyelia) causes loss of pain and temperature sensation bilaterally over local segments — suspended dissociated sensory loss (see Figure 1.47).

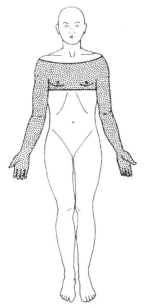

Figure 1.47 Suspended area of dissociated sensory loss (to pain and temperature only) as seen with a dilated central canal, damaging fibres crossing to the spinothalamic tract at their segments of entry (see Figures 1.45 and 1.46).

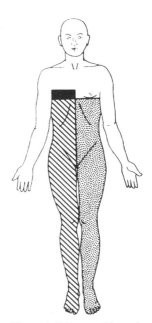

Figure 1.49 Brown–Séquard syndrome due to damage to one side of the spinal cord. While all modalities (black) may be affected at the level of the lesion, joint position sense is affected ipsilaterally (stripes) and pain and temperature sense contralaterally, below the lesion (dots) (see Figure 1.48).

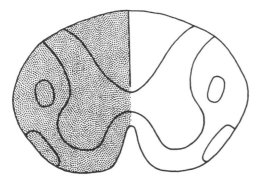

Figure 1.48 Damage to one side of the cord causes ipsilateral weakness and position sense loss and contralateral pain and temperature loss below the lesion (see Figure 1.49).

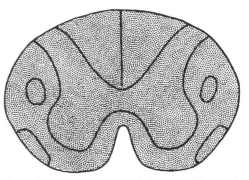

Figure 1.50 Damage to the whole cord with paraplegia and loss of all modalities of sensation is characteristic of transverse myelitis or severe spinal trauma.

sensory level. Levels adjudged on motor or reflex criteria such as focal wasting in the hand (T1) with a paraparesis below were more accurate.

Isolated dorsal column loss leads to position sense loss in the legs, particularly as seen in tabes dorsalis (Figure 1.51) in which the

patients are liable to fall when they close their eyes or when lighting is poor. A combination of dorsal column damage and corticospinal tract impairment is seen in B_{12} deficiency (subacute combined degeneration of the cord) (Figure 1.52). There may often be additional distal sensory loss due to peri-

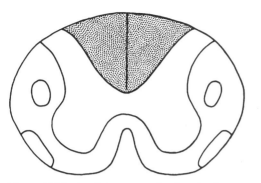

Figure 1.51 Isolated damage to the dorsal columns causes loss of position sense with ataxia, worse in the dark as in tabes dorsalis.

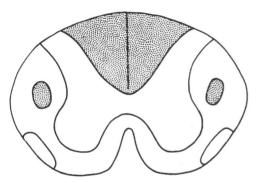

Figure 1.52 Vitamin B$_{12}$ deficiency causes subacute combined degeneration of the cord with upper motor neurone signs and joint position sense loss.

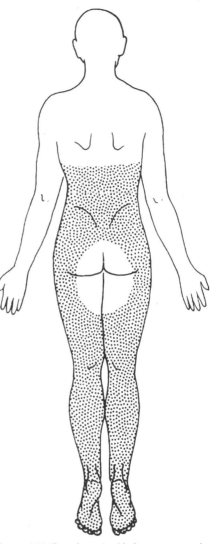

Figure 1.53 'Sacral sparing' below a sensory level due to an intrinsic spinal cord lesion.

pheral neuropathy in this condition. A similar combination with scoliosis and pes cavus is seen in the hereditary condition Friedreich's ataxia, in which progressive ataxia begins in the teens.

As the spinothalamic fibres are arranged in the cord it is possible for a cord lesion, especially an intrinsic one, to spare those that entered first in the sacral region and which lie most superficially. This leads to the phenomenon of 'sacral sparing' in which sensation is lost below a level on the trunk but appreciation of pinprick is 'spared', i.e. preserved over the buttock and perianal region. This is another pattern indicative of a cord lesion (Figure 1.53).

Lesions of the cauda equina produce sensory loss in the lower limbs and over the buttocks and perineum. If only lower sacral dermatomes are affected, for example with a low lumbar central disc prolapse, then the patient may be 'sitting on his physical signs', an adage that recalls the importance of turning the patient over to test the back of the legs and buttocks (Figure 1.54).

The sensory loss of root or peripheral nerve lesions is anatomically distinct and can be seen on the familiar body maps (Figures 1.55–1.76).

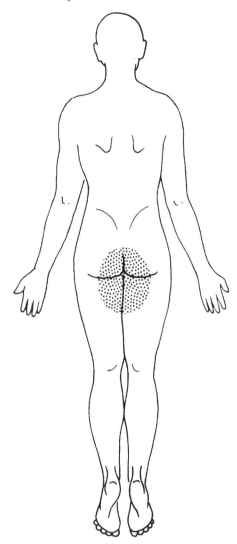

Figure 1.54 Perineal area of sensory loss with a cauda equina lesion.

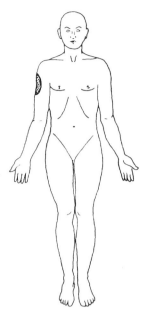

Figure 1.55 Circumflex nerve. The small patch on the outer arm is affected. It may be seen in context of neuralgic amyotrophy or after the brachial plexus is affected by immunization.

In the hand there is often a problem distinguishing the cause of sensory disturbances. They may be seen with hemisphere problems (e.g. tumours or ischaemia), with root entry zone plaques in multiple sclerosis, with root lesions from cervical spondylosis, with plexus damage (e.g. by a cervical rib), or with the carpal tunnel syndrome or ulnar neuritis. The sensory loss may be global in the hand with astereognosis with the central lesion, accompanied by severe joint position sense

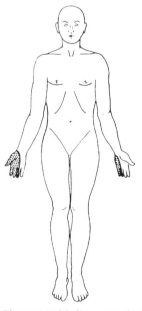

Figure 1.56 Median nerve (right hand) and ulnar nerve (left hand) lesions affect $3\frac{1}{2}$ and $1\frac{1}{2}$ fingers, respectively.

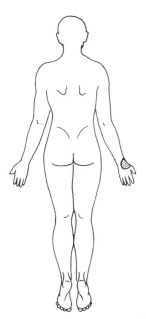

Figure 1.57 Radial nerve palsies may appear not to affect sensation but the area over the anatomical snuffbox at the base of the thumb on the back of the hand may be affected.

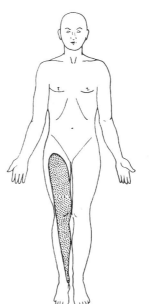

Figure 1.59 Femoral nerve lesion. The medial side of the knee and shin is the most constant area of disturbance (note similarity with L3–4 dermatomes) (see Figures 1.69 and 1.70).

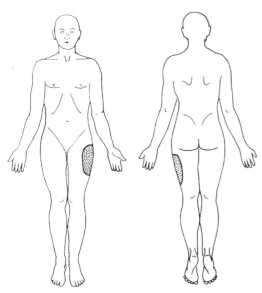

Figure 1.58 Lateral cutaneous nerve of the thigh: the area on the lateral aspect of the thigh is the size of the patient's hand and is affected in 'meralgia paraesthetica'.

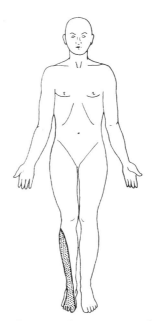

Figure 1.60 Common peroneal nerve lesion. The area affected may be restricted to the lower part of the shaded area.

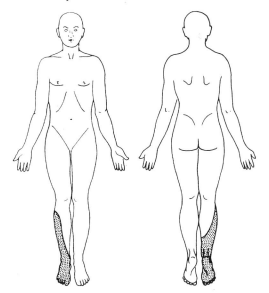

Figure 1.61 Sciatic nerve lesion with sensory disturbances over the common peroneal and sural nerve territories.

Sensory dematones

C6

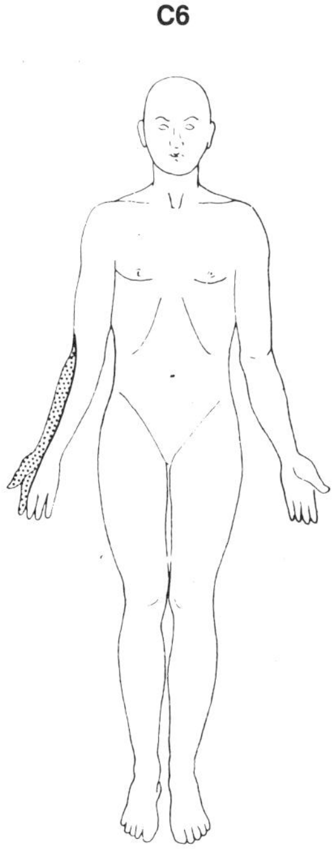

Figure 1.63 Sensory loss of root lesion at C6.

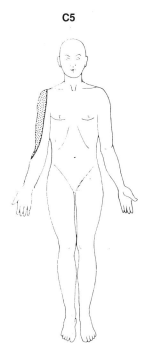

C5

Figure 1.62 Sensory loss of root lesion at C5.

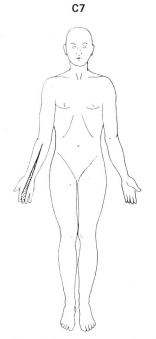

C7

Figure 1.64 Sensory loss of root lesion at C7.

C8

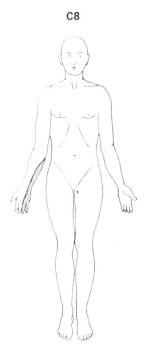

Figure 1.65 Sensory loss of root lesion at C8.

L1

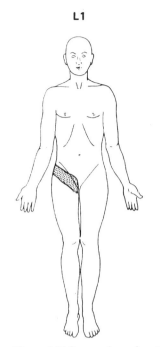

Figure 1.67 Sensory loss of root lesion at L1.

T1

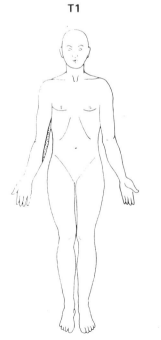

Figure 1.66 Sensory loss of root lesion at T1.

L2

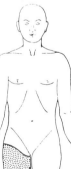
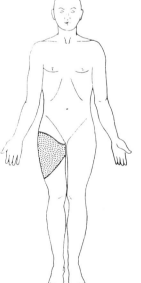

Figure 1.68 Sensory loss of root lesion at L2.

L3

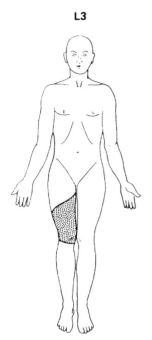

Figure 1.69 Sensory loss of root lesion at L3.

L5

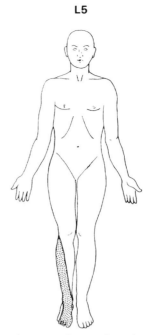

Figure 1.71 Sensory loss of root lesion at L5.

L4

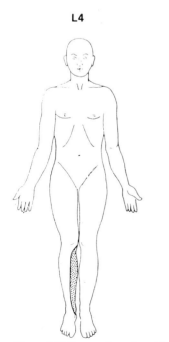

Figure 1.70 Sensory loss of root lesion at L4.

S1

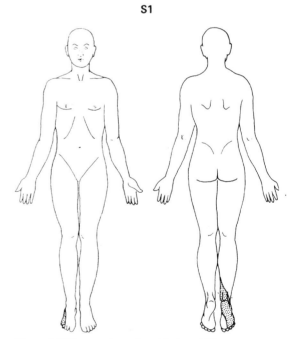

Figure 1.72 Sensory loss of root lesion at S1.

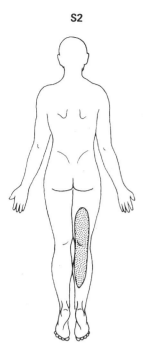

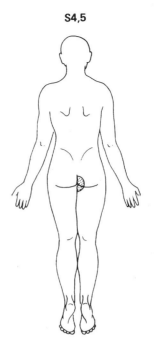

Figure 1.73 Sensory loss of root lesion at S2.

Figure 1.75 Sensory loss of root lesion at S4–5.

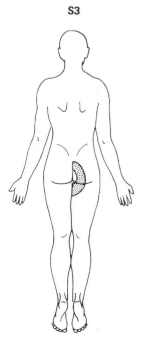

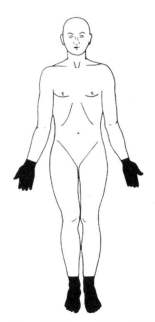

Figure 1.74 Sensory loss of root lesion at S3.

Figure 1.76 Loss of all modalities in glove and stocking distribution due a peripheral neuropathy.

loss if it is in the dorsal root entry zone or selective within the hand if due to root or peripheral nerve lesions. Sensory symptoms in the thumb and index may be due to the carpal tunnel syndrome, when the only loss will be distal to the wrist (Figure 1.56) and indeed often restricted to impaired two-point discrimination in the index. If due to a C6 root lesion, the impairment will also be demonstrated on the lateral border of the forearm (Figure 1.63). If symptoms are felt in the medial two fingers, the loss may be in the little finger and half the ring finger and not extend above the wrist crease if due to an ulnar lesion (Figure 1.56), but involve both fingers and the medial border of the forearm if due to a C8–T1 lesion such as is caused by a cervical rib (Figure 1.65).

Root sensory loss may also be revealed by testing joint position sense. The patient's complaint of a clumsy or numb hand may prove to be associated with loss of joint position sense in the thumb (C6), middle finger (C7) or little finger (C8). If joint position sense loss is more marked in the fingers than in the toes, a lesion affecting the dorsal columns at the foramen magnum should be suspected. Severe joint position sense loss leads to a wavering instability of the fingers, a kind of involuntary movement referred to as pseudo-athetosis.

Normally, attention to the maps will enable the examiner to determine the origin of a patch of sensory loss but it should be realized that these maps are the median of a range. Patients differ in detail and slightly atypical dermatomes or peripheral nerve territories may be encountered.

Peripheral neuropathy causes either patchy sensory loss due to involvement of many individual nerves (mononeuritis multiplex) or a distal glove and stocking loss. Patients with peripheral neuropathy complain of paraesthesiae and blunting of sensation in their extremities, and may also say that they are walking on cotton wool. They may also have pain in their calves. Pinprick may appear blunt as it is tested from below upwards until reaching say mid-calf or above the wrist. Cotton-wool touches may be missed in the hands and feet though detected accurately over the forearm or thigh. Vibration sense may be impaired at the toes but normal at the knees. The sensory changes of a peripheral neuropathy are thus in the periphery (Figure 1.76). The peripheral nerves should be palpated as thickening suggests recurrent demyelination and remyelination of nerves as in hereditary neuropathies and leprosy. Autonomic damage may be suggested by dryness of the hands and feet, due to loss of sweating, sensitivity to bright light due to paralysis of pupil reflexes, and postural dizziness due to postural hypotension. Loss of beat-to-beat variation of the pulse during deep breathing, a blocked Valsalva response, and a neurogenic bladder and impotence are other features seen when autonomic fibres are affected.

Further reading

MEDICAL RESEARCH COUNCIL (1990) *Aids to the Examination of the Peripheral Nervous System*. Baillière Tindall, London.
STEWART, J.D. (1993) *Focal Peripheral Neuropathies*, 2nd edn. Raven Press, New York.

The unconscious patient

The first priority when approaching this problem is to secure an adequate airway and ventilation, and to support the circulation if necessary. Then attention can be focused on the diagnostic questions of whether coma is due to metabolic depression of neuronal function, a diffuse disease such as meningitis, or whether it follows from the effects of a focal structural lesion in the brain. The responsible lesion may be in the reticular substance of the brain stem which is normally responsible for maintaining the alert state of the cerebrum through its tonic activity (Figure 1.77), or it can be the result of mechanical distortion and squeezing of the brain stem from an expanding mass elsewhere in the skull (Figure 1.78).

The examination of the nervous system has to be modified to sort out these different pos-

national use is that of the Glasgow Coma Scale (Table 1.17). This simply describes the level of responsiveness as judged by eye opening, speech and movement to simple stimuli like the spoken word, and pain. Deterioration is readily detected and the scale proves 'robust' in practice, little error resulting from the use of different examiners at sequential examinations.

It is also important to be able to detect the hemiparesis that may be a clue to a possible hemisphere mass lesion causing coma by displacing structures, which is potentially lethal. Facial weakness on one side is shown by the blowing out of one cheek during expiration, or by an asymmetry of grimace in response to painful stimuli. Asymmetry of the limbs is then sought. The upper limb may be flat on the sheet, the leg extended and externally rotated on the hemiparetic side. The amount of spontaneous movement can be revealing, as can the way the limb falls back on to the bed when lifted and released. The flaccid hemiplegic side falls more like a dead weight than the more normal side. Finally, the response to pain is watched. The arm may move purposefully to the site of the pain, or flex, or go into an extended internally rotated decerebrate posture. If one arm flexes but the other extends, the latter more primitive response is

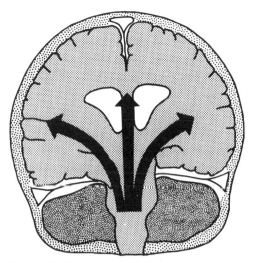

Figure 1.77 The reticular formation of the brain stem maintains the conscious state of the cerebral hemispheres.

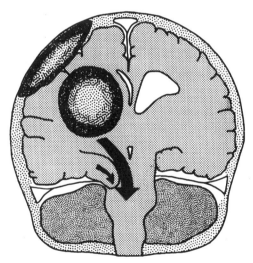

Figure 1.78 Herniation of the temporal lobe onto the third cranial nerve (small arrow) or pressure on the brain stem (large arrow) cause the signs associated with an increasing mass lesion whether extracerebral or intracerebral.

sibilities. First and foremost a measure of the depth of coma is desirable as deterioration may mean support of ventilation is about to become necessary, and also raises the possibility of the progressive effects of a remediable mass lesion. The system in widespread inter-

Table 1.17 Glasgow Coma Scale

Eye opening	
Spontaneous	4
To speech	3
To pain	2
Nil	1
Verbal response	
Orientated	5
Confused conversation	4
Inappropriate words	3
Incomprehensible sounds	2
Nil	1
Best motor response	
Obeys	6
Localizes	5
Withdraws	4
Abnormal flexion	3
Extension response	2
Nil	1

indicative of a hemiparesis on that side. Arm responses are concentrated upon as spinal pathology and reflex activity may affect those in the legs unrelated to cerebral changes. The most useful painful stimulus to judge the symmetry of response is in the midline. The knuckles of the examiner's clenched fist are rolled on the sternum whilst exerting firm pressure. This technique also avoids the problem of hemisensory loss distorting the response on one side. It may be necessary also to use a cranial stimulus, for example after head injury when a cervical cord injury may also have occurred, causing a loss of pain appreciation below the neck. Pressure with a thumb over either supraorbital nerve at the orbital ridge is the best manoeuvre. Some press on the styloid process instead. Repeated stimulation of the limbs may leave bruises which are distressing so rather than pinching the loose skin on the inside of the arm as is often advised, it is better to squeeze the nail bed, perhaps with the side of a pencil.

Most important in the neurological examination of the unconscious patient is the assessment of brain-stem functions. To this end pupil reflexes, eye movements and respiratory patterns are observed. The conditions are often not ideal for seeing if the pupils react. The patient is usually in a well-lit area, often in the open plan of an Intensive Care Unit. It is important to produce some shading and to use a very bright testing light. A normal response of the pupils implies integrity of the brain stem, making it likely that the coma is due to some metabolic or diffuse process and not to a local cause. Interpretation is made impossible if the patient has had drugs that paralyse the pupil response, e.g. scopolamine, or the patient has been anoxic, when the pupils may be large and fixed. Drug overdose classically produces coma with preserved pupil responses.

Eye movement can be induced in the unconscious patient in one of two ways. Firstly, the head can be rolled from one side to the other, which triggers the normal vestibulo-ocular reflex which produces counter-rolling eye movements. This manoeuvre is not to be used in a head injured patient in case there is also cervical cord damage. If this proves an inadequate stimulus the external auditory meatus should be syringed with ice-cold water; 40–50 ml are injected with an ordinary plastic syringe. If the brain stem is intact, conjugate gaze develops towards the irrigated ear on either side. If the brain stem has been damaged by an intrinsic lesion, or by compression, there may be unilateral loss of conjugate gaze, or the induced movements may be dysconjugate, e.g. abduction of one eye without matching adduction of the other eye. Total loss of movements also implies pontine damage unless the patient is in very deep coma (obvious from the depressed state of respiration and hypotonic arreflexic immobility, for example after massive barbiturate overdose). Symmetrical divergence of the eyes at rest is not of diagnostic importance.

Respiration may be simply depressed, for example by drug overdose, or an abnormal pattern of movements may develop. The gradual progression from deep breaths to shallow ones or a pause and back again (Cheyne–Stokes respiration) may occur with either metabolic or diffuse diseases or from early brain stem compression, so it is of little diagnostic help. Other patterns of so-called ataxic breathing, apneustic breathing, inspiratory pauses, etc., imply brain-stem dysfunction. Regular deep breaths suggest ketosis. The breath may smell of alcohol or of ketones, and some observers claim to be able to detect characteristic changes in liver disease and renal failure.

Armed with information about any change in the level of consciousness, pupil reactions, eye movement and motor responses, it is usually possible to deduce the type of coma: whether due to metabolic or diffuse processes or primary or secondary brain-stem damage. Stable or lightening coma with depressed but regular respiration and preserved pupil responses, intact eye movements and symmetrical hypotonic limbs is characteristic of metabolic coma or that due to disease such as meningitis. Metabolic conditions are also suggested if there are mismatches, for example between severe respiratory depression with preserved spontaneous limb movements.

Brain-stem lesions causing coma are recognizable by abnormalities of pupil response and eye movements, and bilateral long tract signs. Intrinsic lesions such as infarcts or haemorrhages cause such abnormalities from the outset. Brain-stem compression by a hemisphere mass lesion also causes loss of pupil reflexes and abnormal patterns of eye movement but these develop *pari passu* with a declining level of consciousness (Table 1.18) whilst under observation. A supratentorial mass lesion may also cause a third nerve palsy by provoking herniation of the temporal lobe over the free edge of the tentorial shelf onto the third nerve. This is manifested by dilatation of the pupil followed by loss of movements as revealed by counterrolling of the head or caloric stimulation. The appearance of a third nerve palsy and/or sequential loss of brain-stem function is, therefore, the hallmark of a mass lesion and should be seen as the indication to refer the patient for urgent neurosurgical advice.

In practice, drug overdose and metabolic disturbances are the commonest causes (about two-thirds), with supratentorial and infratentorial structural lesions accounting for about one-sixth of cases each. In the distinction of metabolic causes, the patient's colour may be helpful. Pallor may be seen with shock or anaemia, a cherry-red colour with carbon monoxide poisoning and a yellow tinge with hepatic failure. Sweating suggests hypoglycaemia when not due to shock. Slow relaxing tendon jerks and low body temperature suggest hypothermia. There are usually signs of the background disease when coma is due to cardiorespiratory failure, uraemia, diabetes, or hepatic failure. Hyponatremia and hypercalcaemia also need to be sought. Very small pupils may be a sign of morphia abuse (but are also seen with pontine haemorrhage). Bilateral extensor plantars are of no help except in excluding psychogenic unresponsiveness.

The fact that someone has suffered a head injury is usually obvious with facial or scalp lacerations, black eyes, boggy swellings over fracture sites, etc. The differential diagnosis may need to include subarachnoid haemorrhage and an epileptic fit in which the patient has sustained a head injury. A Medilert bracelet or the gum changes of chronic phenytoin ingestion may provide the answer. Another situation that confuses the assessment of the head injury is when the victim is drunk. Measuring blood alcohol levels may be helpful, since coma is likely to be due to the head trauma and not the alcohol, unless the blood level is over 200 mg per 100 ml.

When examining a patient for signs of the sequelae of head injury it is also necessary to consider the possibility of coincident spinal trauma. A stiff neck may be due to subarachnoid bleeding caused by the head injury but may be a pointer to local damage, and a full set of cervical spine films should be obtained in all cases of head injury with impaired consciousness. A discrepancy in movement between the upper and lower limbs should also prompt full examination and X-ray study of the rest of the spine. Facial injury in a fall, or a report that the patient was found prone, should raise suspicions of hyperextension injury to the neck.

Locked-in syndrome

Ventral damage in the pons may rob the patient of the ability to speak, move his limbs or any muscle supplied by lower cranial

Table 1.18 Progressive changes of tentorial herniation

Stage	Pupils	Eyes (position and counter-rolling movements)	Respiration	Motor signs
1	Small reacting	Roving or central Loss of reflex upgaze	Sighs, yawns, Cheyne–Stokes	Extensor plantars
2	Medium fixed	Dysconjugate reflex movements	Hyperventilation	Decerebrate
3	Medium fixed	No reflex movements	Regular rapid	Flaccid
4	Dilated fixed	No reflex movements	Slow gasping	Flaccid

nerves. This total lack of ability to communi-
cate may be misinterpreted as impaired
awareness. The patient's eyes are open, however, and often the patient can indicate his
responsiveness by a blink or a vertical eye
movement. If the locked-in state is suspected
the patient should be asked to blink to order
and then to blink once for 'yes' and twice for
'no' in order to carry out an albeit limited
'conversation'. An EEG will confirm the
patient's responsiveness to environmental stimuli. The cause is usually vascular and often
fatal but occasionally recovery is possible.
Clearly this state must always be excluded
lest distressing remarks are made over a
patient who is not in coma.

Coma vigil (akinetic mutism)

Here some degree of vigilance is suspected
because the patient may have open eyes
which appear to follow visual targets, but in
truth the patient is not alert. They vocalize
little if at all, and are doubly incontinent.
Noxious stimuli produce little or no response.
This state may be due to bilateral frontal lobe
infarction or the diffuse effects of hypoxia,
hypoglycaemia, head injury or hydrocephalus.
Disturbance of the reticular formation is the
usual substratum. There are some superficial
similarities with the locked-in syndrome, but
no communication can be established with the
patient suffering from akinetic mutism, and
the EEG shows no reaction to external stimuli.

Chronic vegetative state

After some severe head injuries, even though
no recovery of higher function occurs, some
patients' coma changes in that cycles of sleep
and wakefulness appear. The patients may or
may not be akinetic. Their eyes may open to
verbal stimuli but no communication is possible. As respiration is well maintained, prolonged survival is possible. At post mortem
the brain stem is relatively spared but there
is extensive damage to the cortex and fore-
brain.

Further reading

BATES, D. (1985) Predicting recovery from medical coma. *Br.
J. Hosp. Med.*, **33**, 276.

FISHER, C.M. (1977) The neurological examination of the
comatose patient. *Acta Neurol. Scand.*, **36**, suppl. 1.

PLUM, F. and POSNER, J.B. (1980) *The Diagnosis of Stupor and
Coma*, 3rd edn. F.A. Davis, Philadelphia.

Brain death

The brain-dead patient is a product of modern
medicine. Mechanical ventilation and support
of the circulation may allow a heart beat to
continue after the patient's brain is irretriev-
ably damaged. If this state of affairs can be
recognized, distressing and unhelpfully protracted efforts at resuscitation can be avoided
and transplant organs of good quality
obtained. The pre-condition for a diagnosis
of brain death is the identification of brain
damage of an irreversible nature, e.g. cerebral
haemorrhage or head injury.

In those circumstances the clinical demonstration of total failure of the brain stem is
sufficient to predict with total confidence
that recovery cannot occur. To this end, it is

Table 1.19 Brain death criteria

Preconditions
Positively diagnosed cause of irreversible structural
brain damage
Absence of complicating hypothermia, metabolic
derangement or drug effect (muscle relaxants,
respiratory depressants, sedation)

Criteria
Unresponsiveness, except spinal reflexes
Apnoea, in absence of prior hyperventilation
Fixed pupils, no eye movement, in absence of ototoxic
drugs or vestibular damage
Loss corneal, gag, swallowing and cough reflexes

Confirmatory tests (not essential)
Isoelectric EEG
Lack of cerebral blood flow

important to show that pupils are fixed to a bright light, that there are no eye movements during ice-cold water irrigation of the ears, that corneal, gag, cough and swallowing reflexes are absent and that the patient is apnoeic. Gag, cough and swallowing reflexes are easily judged when carrying out tracheal toilet. Testing for apnoea requires care. The patient must not be endangered, so should be ventilated with oxygen prior to looking for evidence of respiratory movements off the respirator. Oxygen via a tracheal cannula at 6 l/min can further protect against anoxia. The essence of the test is that $paCO_2$ rises off the ventilator and produces a stimulus to respiratory neurones. It follows that the $paCO_2$ must be normal at the beginning of the period of observation and not low due to over-ventilation. This can either be checked by arterial blood gas sampling, or 5% CO_2 can be added to the inspired air for 5 minutes before switching off the ventilator.

It is essential when assessing the results of these tests to exclude the effects of drugs or hypothermia. If there is any doubt, time must be allowed to elapse for elimination of any pharmacological agents.

Further reading

PALLIS, C. and HARLEY D. (1996) *ABC of Brain Stem Death*, 2nd edn. British Medical Journal, London.

2

Common problems

Headache

The problem with headache (Figure 2.1) is that it is a commonplace symptom that may be of no medical significance but it can also be the first manifestation of a lethal or disabling disease. The patient's own fears about the cause of the headache not only affect the likelihood of seeking advice but also contaminate the history. If the first medical attendant shrugs off the problem there is a risk the headache may become 'continuous' or more 'severe' or accompanied by dizziness, when related to the second observer. It is, therefore, important that the first history is sympathetically and carefully taken, and this requires time.

Sudden headache

A headache of abrupt onset (Figure 2.2), perhaps described by the patient with a snap of their fingers, or as if struck on the head, is characteristic of a sudden event such as bleed-

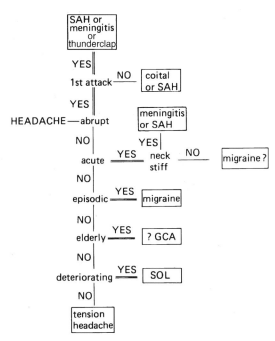

Figure 2.1 Flow chart for the diagnosis of headache. SAH = subarachnoid haemorrhage; GCA = giant cell arteritis; SOL = space-occupying lesion.

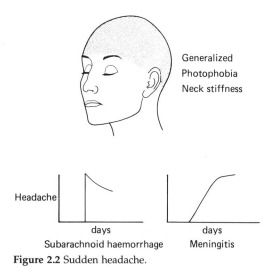

Figure 2.2 Sudden headache.

ing into the subarachnoid space. In this circumstance, vomiting is also common and the patient develops a stiff neck. Admission for a diagnostic lumbar puncture and/or CT scan is necessary. If these tests reveal no evidence of intracranial bleeding and the headache does not persist, the probability is that this is what has been called a thunderclap headache, which proves benign. At the moment of sexual climax, some individuals develop a sudden throbbing generalized headache (coital cephalagia) which also usually proves benign and appears to be akin to a migrainous event.

Continuous headache

Most patients with continuous, all-day, every-day headache will have tension headaches (Figure 2.3). This can be confidently assumed when the history dates back a matter of years and the complaint is of a sense of pressure at the vertex or a tight band. When the story is only a few months old, however, other possibilities need consideration. In the elderly, giant cell arteritis must always be considered and a confirmatory ESR carried out there and then. There may be scalp tenderness, malaise and jaw claudication and the temporal vessels may be tender, nodular or occluded. The

headache is again throbbing in nature. Its temporal localization can cause confusion with temporomandibular joint disease.

The headache due to a cerebral tumour (Figure 2.4) may be continuous but the most suspicious features are increasing severity, associated symptoms implying neurological dysfunction, or change of the headache in circumstances that raise intracranial pressure (straining, bending over, lying down). The pain may be described as 'bursting'. Other less sinister headaches such as migraine may be aggravated by head jolt, a cough or sneeze, however. Obstructions of vision with exercise or change of posture imply the presence of critical optic nerve perfusion due to the presence of papilloedema, so add to the sinister sound of a headache. The headache of raised intracranial pressure is often present on waking, but so too is that of depression.

The site of the headache may help locate the responsible mass lesion. The pain-sensitive structures in the head are the blood vessels and the dura. Pain tends to be referred to the territory of the sensory nerve supplying the affected dura. Thus pain arising in the anterior fossa is often felt in the forehead (1st division trigeminal nerve). Middle fossa lesions may produce pain under the ipsilateral eye (2nd division trigeminal nerve). Convexity lesions produce headache felt at the vertex or over the parietal or temporal area. Posterior fossa mass lesions tend to cause pain in the occiput, neck or rarely the shoulder, throat or behind

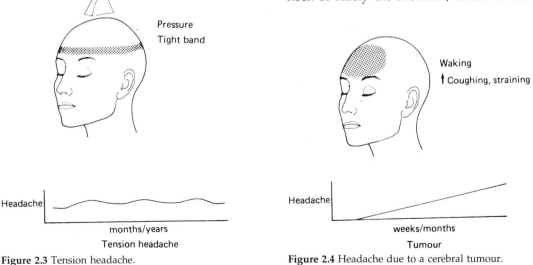

Figure 2.3 Tension headache.

Figure 2.4 Headache due to a cerebral tumour.

the mastoid. Headache of this type in a young obese female with papilloedema but no neurological findings on examination, suggests the diagnosis of benign intracranial hypertension. This may be seen in individuals receiving tetracycline, coming off steroids, with hypervitaminosis A, or who have intracranial venous sinus thrombosis.

Rapidly developing headache

Severe headache coming on over a day or two may prove to be the first of many such events and so classifiable as migrainous, but may also be seen with meningitis (see Figure 2.2). The meningitic patient is usually ill, febrile and found to have neck stiffness but a lumbar puncture may have to be done without these supportive features being present if there have not been previous similar episodes indicative of migraine.

Periodic headache

An occasional severe headache, lasting a few hours, is commonly due to migraine (Figure 2.5). Classical migraine attacks involve visual disturbance, often an evolving enlarging crescent of scintillating zig-zag lines, perhaps in

hemianopic distribution, or hemisensory phenomena. These appear to be due to a distinct entity. Other periodic headaches associated with nausea or dizziness are less certainly due to a definable condition. Computer searches of the histories given by headache sufferers reveal instead a spectrum from periodic bilious headaches ('migraine') at one end, to the continuous tight band due to tension at the other. The practical conclusion is that stressful circumstances are relevant throughout the spectrum and that mixed headaches due to tension and migraine commonly occur. Migraine attacks may be accompanied by a small or dilated pupil, a full 3rd nerve palsy or even a hemiparesis, which is at risk of becoming persistent if the sufferer is also on the contraceptive pill.

Although textbooks suggest migraine always causes unilateral throbbing headache, 50% have bilateral headache and the pain may be continuous during the attack. The headache may be ipsilateral to any limb weakness or sensory disturbance. Some patients observe that attacks are precipitated by their periods, weekends, certain foods, alcohol, exercise, heading a football, missed meals, the contraceptive pill, high altitude or vasodilator agents used for angina. It is always worth asking about the effect of alcohol, since it aggravates migraine but relieves tension headaches. Nausea is usual, vomiting common and diarrhoea occasional. Migraine is often better during pregnancy.

The headache of hypertension is generalized or maximal in the occipital area, where it may be present on waking. If the patient has papilloedema due to retinopathy then the distinction from a cerebral tumour can be difficult and CT scanning is advised. The papilloedema of hypertensive retinopathy is normally distinguishable by the florid haemorrhage and exudates well out in the fundus. Haemorrhage in the papilloedematous fundus due to a cerebral tumour is usually less dramatic and located close to the disc. It should be stressed that most headaches associated with arterial hypertension are due to anxiety and follow the patient's learning that he has high blood pressure. Headache causally related to undiagnosed hypertension is said to occur in as few as 10% of cases.

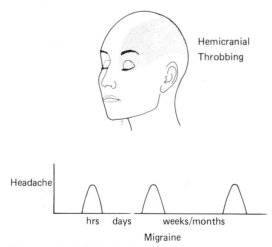

Figure 2.5 Periodic headache due to migraine.

Cervical spondylosis frequently causes neck and suboccipital headache (Figure 2.6), but it may also cause pain over one eye. The clue to the diagnosis comes from the association of pain to bad head posture, the presence of local cervical tenderness and the relief from local heat or massage or the wearing of a collar.

Rarely, glaucoma causes frontal headaches and vomiting that may raise suspicions of a brain tumour. There is usually a complaint of haloes around objects like street lights in the rain, increasing pain when the pupil dilates in the dark, tenderness of the globe and a prominent deep cup in the optic disc on ophthalmoscopy. Urgent ophthalmological attention is required.

Carotid artery disease may cause headache or pain in the neck over the vessel if it occludes. Pain may be referred to the peri-orbital region, however, and there may be a mild ptosis and small pupil due to a Horner's syndrome due to damage to the sympathetic plexus in the wall of the artery.

Some patients develop a severe headache during sexual intercourse. When this has not occurred before, there is a tendency for a sub-arachnoid haemorrhage to be suspected and it may be necessary to investigate such first events to reassure the patient and his medical attendants.

Sinusitis can cause pain over the cheek or frontal region. Bending down often increases the pain. Nose blowing may exacerbate or relieve the pain, there may be local tenderness, and the patient has nasal symptoms. Chronic sinusitis is not considered to be a cause of protracted headache.

Further reading

LANCE, J.W. (1993) *Mechanism and Management of Headache*, 5th edn. Butterworth-Heinemann, London.

Attacks of loss of consciousness

If the patient describes an episode of loss of consciousness not due to head injury, the immediate concern is always, is it epilepsy? The usual result of this anxiety is a rapidly arranged consultation at which the patient arrives without an eyewitness account of the event. It is both cheaper and more effective to request that a witness come to the clinic or writes an account of the episode, than to embark on extensive investigation in the first instance. The EEG is useful in characterizing epilepsy and detecting a clinically unsuspected focus of origin but is poor at answering the question 'was last week's black-out a fit or not?' The diagnosis of epilepsy is always a clinical one, dependent on the details of what happened to the patient before, during, and after the period of altered awareness or behaviour. The crucial questions to have answered by an eyewitness are listed in Table 2.1. The separation between syncope due to brief global cerebral ischaemia as perfusion pressure falls due to cardiac irregularity, hypotension or vagal activity and epilepsy, is indicated. If the situation is unclear it is important not to apply a hasty 'label' to the patient or over-react to the EEG and embark on potentially unnecessary medication. It is better to 'wait and see'.

Patients, especially young ones, who lose consciousness only when upright, who feel

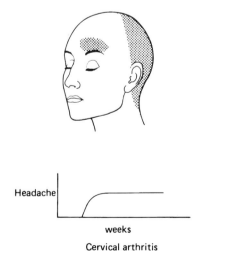

Headache | weeks

Cervical arthritis

Figure 2.6 Headache caused by cervical spondylosis.

Table 2.1 Features of epilepsy and syncope

	Epilepsy	*Syncope*
History of attack		
Warning	In 50% though often indescribable	Usual, 'faint', blurred vision – darkening, tinnitus
Onset	Sudden	Avoidable by change posture, less abrupt
Features	Eyes open Rigidity Convulsed	Eyes closed Limp Minor twitching at most
Examination		
Colour	Pale	Pale
Corneals	Lost	Intact
Plantars	Extensor	Flexor
History of aftermath		
Recovery	Confused, headache, sleepy	'Washed out', sweating, 'cold and clammy'
Examination		
Prolactin	Rises 20 mins after major attack	Unchanged

faint with ringing in the ears and blackening vision before slumping limply to the ground for up to a couple of minutes with no movements, or incontinence, and recovering with marked sweating, are easily recognized as having suffered from syncope. Their colour will have drained, they will have looked cold and clammy and on recovery, though 'exhausted' and perhaps nauseated, they will not be confused.

By contrast, a sudden loss of consciousness when lying down, heralded by a cry, with eyes open, stiffening then shaking of the limbs, self-injury and incontinence followed on recovery by confusion, headache and a desire to sleep is clearly due to epilepsy. If the end of the attack is witnessed, corneal and pupillary reflexes may be impaired and the plantar responses extensor. Pulse and blood pressure are elevated, and the patient may be hypoxic and develop hyperkalaemia, and even rhabdomyolysis. Self injury may include tongue or cheek biting, the fall may have caused head injury, the convulsion may leave the patient with muscle pain or even a crush fracture of a vertebra.

The distinction is often difficult, however. While doubt is usually due to incomplete information, there are often confusing aspects of the history. Some patients who faint may be incontinent if their bladder was full at the time, some keep their eyes open, and even have multifocal myoclonic jerks. Some may pass out in the sitting position and others, if prevented from falling, may go on to a tonic convulsion with brief stiffening and minor twitching of the extremities. Such episodes have produced alarm and a diagnosis of epilepsy in personal cases where the patient has fainted from heat and fluid loss due to diarrhoea whilst strapped into an aeroplane seat, or propped up in a car seat (by a helpful doctor in the back seat!).

Sudden loss of consciousness out of the blue is always very suspicious of epilepsy and is sometimes the only clue if the attack was not witnessed. Temporal lobe attacks have their own characteristic story. The patient may have an epigastric rising sensation, a hallucination of smell, taste, sight or sound or make lip-smacking or grimacing expressions. In epileptic fugues the patient may go through the motions of making a meal, or travelling on public transport with no awareness or recall later. Sometimes the complaint is of the slow or fast passing of time. Deja vu and less often jamais vu experiences can be epileptic, but a rare deja vu feeling can be normal. Others describe attacks of fear or anger. A personal case brought a letter torn into small pieces. When this was laboriously reconstituted it read 'subject to outbursts of rage'. The distinction between epileptic and psychological outbursts depends on the sudden onset and offset of epileptic events. The patient may make semi-purposeful movements, e.g. picking at their clothes, or whistle or mutter. As amnesia of the content of the attack is common, these features may only be remembered hazily. Such attacks last about 90 seconds.

Petit mal is a distinct entity with onset in childhood. The attacks consist of a brief 'absence' when the child stares blankly and is inaccessible. The eyelids flutter but any other movement is unusual. The EEG is diagnostic (Table 2.2). The attack lasts about 10–12

Table 2.2 Types of epilepsy

International classification	Old clinical classification	Main features
I. PARTIAL SEIZURES		
(a) With elementary symptomatology (generally without impaired consciousness)	Focal (Jacksonian)	Spreading jactitation of limb or face, spreading sensory disturbance limb or face
(b) With complex symptomatology (generally with impaired consciousness)	Psychomotor (temporal lobe)	Epigastric rising sensation, smell or taste hallucination, visual or auditory hallucination, lip smacking, grimace, automatic behaviour, amnesia for event
(c) Secondarily generalized	Focal becoming generalized	Jacksonian or psychomotor attack going on to grand mal
II. GENERALIZED SEIZURES including petit mal	Petit mal	Childhood onset, simple 'absence' 10–15 seconds 3 Hz spike and wave discharge on EEG
Tonic-clonic	Grand mal	Childhood or adult onset tonic, clonic, or tonic followed by clonic seizure, cyanosis, self-injury, incontinence followed by confusion and headache
Akinetic	Lennox–Gastaut	Age 1–6, drop attacks, brief tonic spells with irregular spike and wave EEG
Infantile spasms	Hypsarrythmia	Infancy, brief flexor spasms (salaams) accompanied by high-voltage disorganized EEG
III. UNILATERAL SEIZURES		Features of generalized seizure, e.g. tonic-clonic but asymmetrical limb involvement
IV. UNCLASSIFIED (data incomplete)		

seconds. The child may be aware of a missed moment or may simply go back to their previous activity as though nothing had happened.

Many little turns prove to be due to temporal lobe discharge rather than petit mal, and elderly patients do not develop petit mal. During the attack the patient's pulse may be raised, the pupils dilated, and there may be increased salivation and sweating. The importance of accurate diagnosis of the type of seizure is the practical one that different drugs are preferred for different types of attack. Focal seizures arising other than in the temporal lobe may produce turning of the head and eyes (adversive seizures arising from either frontal lobe), or a spread of clonic jerking beginning at the angle of the mouth, in the thumb and index or the big toe or a spread of sensory disturbance in a limb ('Jacksonian' epilepsy arising in the motor or sensory cortex) (see Table 2.2). A rhythmic contraction of hand or face every few seconds may be due to epilepsia partialis continuans. A focal onset to an attack may also be suspected if the patient has focal weakness on recovery (Todd's paresis).

Rarely, epileptic attacks are triggered by external events. The commonest is that due to photic stimulation. The flickering light of a television screen may provoke fits in susceptible children. As most of the central field of both eyes needs to be affected to set off a seizure discharge, the attack can be aborted by closing one eye if presenting symptoms are recognized. The risk is reduced by sitting far from a small set, advice rejected by most children. Reading can trigger epilepsy as rarely as can listening to music or even thinking!

Nocturnal attacks may be suspected if the patient wakes with blood on the pillow, in a wet bed or with aching muscles. Parents may hear a cry and find the child in a deep sleep, very difficult to wake, with a sore tongue or cheek when they do finally wake.

The search for a cause for seizures depends on the age of onset. In neonates biochemical causes like hypoglycaemia, hypocalcaemia and hypoxia predominate. In young children the commonest cause is birth injury, but some congenital anomalies or tuberose sclerosis can also be responsible. Febrile fits and those due to meningitis also affect toddlers. In adolescence most attacks are idiopathic with the inference of genetic predisposition. Young adults have often sustained a significant head injury, or have abused drugs or alcohol. Older adults (say, older than 25) are always suspected of harbouring a cerebral tumour. Although tumour is a more likely cause of epilepsy in middle life than at any other time, the yield of investigation is still low unless the fits are focal or the EEG suggests they are focal, or the clinical examination has produced evidence of a hemisphere deficit. One of the problems of investigating such patients is that tumours may provoke a fit before they are large enough to register on scans. A false sense of security may prevail. Such patients should be re-examined and have repeat EEGs and scans if any suspicious features develop. In the elderly, CT scans may reveal cerebral infarcts that have not been clinically overt (as strokes) but appear to be the cause of epilepsy of late onset. MRI scans produce an even higher yield of such infarcts. Interestingly, not all are cortical, though the initial ischaemic episode and scarring may have included the cortex, although the residual visible lesion on the scan may be deeper. Alternatively, such deep infarcts may just be a marker of cerebrovascular disease and its invisible effects (in the cortex) are the cause of fits. Degenerative conditions may also cause seizures in the elderly. Status epilepticus can be due to a new lesion, e.g. a stroke, encephalitis or a tumour, particularly in the frontal lobe, or to lack of compliance with antiepileptic drugs in a patient with long-standing epilepsy.

Withdrawal from alcohol abuse (after an interval of 6–48 hours) can also trigger status, and non-ketotic hyperglycaemia is a rare cause of epilepsia partialis continuans. Hypocalcaemia may cause true fits. Associated depression or other mental disturbance is suggestive of hypocalcaemia and tetanic cramps or paraesthesiae in the extremities confirmative. The diagnosis is clinched by measuring the serum level. Other metabolic causes of fits include hyponatremia, hypoglycaemia, and diabetes insipidus.

Some drugs, like tricyclic antidepressants and phenothiazines, may lower the seizure threshold. An acute dystonic reaction from phenothiazines may alternatively produce a sudden attack of rigidity which may be misconstrued as a seizure.

If syncope is clearly the cause of loss of consciousness, the next step is to try to determine whether this is due to a vasovagal reflex, e.g. at the sight of blood or on a hot day when under stress. For these cases no treatment is needed and simple explanations will enable the patient to look after himself, putting his head between his knees when symptoms begin. Postural fainting suggests postural hypotension due to recent bed rest, over-effective drugs for hypertension or autonomic neuropathy as in diabetes mellitus, amyloidosis, the Shy–Drager syndrome or sometimes after drugs like chlorpromazine or vincristine. A complaint of palpitations or flushing at the end of an attack as blood flow returns to the vasodilated ischaemic tissues suggests a cardiac arrhythmia. ECG abnormalities on routine records or after 24-hour Holter monitoring need to be assessed by experts in their interpretation as not all deviations from normal are of haemodynamic significance. Syncope in middle-aged males may occur when they get up in the night to empty a full bladder (micturition syncope). Paroxysms of coughing in the bronchitic may also lead to syncope.

Hypoglycaemia as a cause of black-outs is readily recognized if attacks occur before breakfast or after missed meals and are accompanied by profuse sweating. The loss of consciousness may last an hour or so, much longer than after a seizure. Confused behaviour often occurs as the blood sugar falls. One case known to the author was found crawling about in the street giving away £5 notes! When the patient is diabetic the possibility of hypoglycaemia comes easily to mind but it should be recalled that epilepsy may be provoked by hypoglycaemia and ongoing epilepsy may result from prior hypoglycaemic brain damage. In the non-diabetic the possibility of a rare insulinoma is suggested by changes in appetite and weight gain. If such hypoglycaemia is suspected, a 72-hour fast may produce symptomatic hypoglycaemia. The simultaneous measurement of blood sugar and serum insulin levels or C peptide may be needed to establish the diagnosis.

Hyperventilation produces feelings of faintness usually short of loss of consciousness and dizziness, usually accompanied by a dry mouth, chest tightness and by paraesthesiae, particularly in the hands and around the mouth. Tetanic cramps of the fingers which are extended with the wrists flexed make the diagnosis clear but usually the clue lies in the patient's statement that when feeling faint he has difficulty taking a deep breath. Eyewitnesses record pallor and distress and may have noticed the sighs and deep breathing. It is worth asking the patient to hyperventilate in the clinic to see if symptoms are reproduced. (This may also usefully provoke petit mal attacks in children.) It may then be enough to explain the mechanism of the panic attack. Some patients benefit from being taught relaxation exercises to give them the confidence to prevent over-breathing. Others need formal psychiatric help.

Loss of consciousness may also occur at the height of headache due to migraine, in an attack of Ménière's disease or with acute obstructive hydrocephalus as produced by the ball-valve effect of a colloid cyst of the third ventricle. In the last situation, weakness of the legs may also develop, suddenly causing falls which can be mistaken for brief fits.

Hysterical fits or pseudoseizures are often very difficult to distinguish. Black-outs that occur only in public are slightly suspect. Pseudoseizures are commoner in young people, in women, and there is some evidence of an increased incidence of abuse in the past. A story of disturbed behaviour for hours on end rarely proves to be due to epilepsy. If attacks are witnessed, and they usually occur in front of medical attendants or nurses, exaggerated movements that put the patient at no risk, a lack of cyanosis, intact corneals and flexor plantar responses all raise doubts about the organic nature of a fit. Bilateral movements without loss of consciousness are suspect. The movements often include side to side movements of the head, and pelvic thrusting of a sexual kind. Prolactin levels do not rise after a pseudoseizure (but do after a major convulsion). An EEG may be entirely normal within minutes of an 'attack'. A special problem arises with epileptic patients who also have pseudoseizures. These seem especially likely to occur when intoxicated with antiepileptic drugs. The complaint of more attacks may lead to an inappropriate further increase in medication if the different nature of the episodes is not realized. In-patient observation may be necessary to sort out how many attacks are pseudoseizures. EEG telemetry and video recording have proved particularly valuable in this situation.

If it is concluded that seizures are occurring, an EEG is indicated to confirm the nature of little attacks as petit mal or temporal lobe epilepsy and to detect a focal source for grand mal. If the attacks are focal or there are focal signs or the EEG contains a focal disturbance, further investigation by CT scanning for the presence of a structural cerebral lesion is indicated. Most physicians would request a CT scan or MRI in any patient whose epilepsy begins after the age of about 25. MRI is particularly useful in the case of temporal lobe epilepsy as it may reveal subtle structural changes, and may indicate if there is a surgical option should drug treatment prove unsatisfactory. Serological tests and the serum calcium are worth checking in all patients with epilepsy except young people with petit mal.

Drug treatment is indicated for most but not all patients.

Further reading

LAIDLAW, J.P., RICHENS, A., CHADWICK, D. (1992) *A Textbook of Epilepsy*, 4th edn. Churchill Livingstone, Edinburgh.

EPILEPSY OCTET (1990) *Lancet*, 336: 93, 161, 231, 291, 350, 423, 486, 551.

KAPOUR, W.N. (1990) Evaluation and outcome of patients with syncope. *Medicine*, **69**, 160–175.

SHORVON, S. (1994) *Status Epilepticus; its Clinical Features and Treatment in Children and Adults*. Cambridge University Press, Cambridge.

Sleep disorders

Medical interest in sleep disorders has been slow to develop despite the fact that, when surveyed, as many as 10–15% of the population report disturbed sleep within the last month. Insomnia predominates and is rarely a neurological problem but daytime drowsiness is a reason for referral.

Excessive daytime sleepiness

A few systemic conditions such as renal failure, alcoholism, and hypothyroidism need to be considered. Rarely, a major neurological illness has drowsiness as a major symptom. This is true of occasional cases of encephalitis, multiple sclerosis, head injury, and brain stem or hypothalamic glioma, all of which are to be recognized by the other features including clear-cut neurological signs.

The two conditions that need particular consideration are narcolepsy and sleep apnoea.

Narcolepsy

Narcolepsy affects young adults, rarely presenting for the first time after the age of 50. It affects about 1 in 3000 in North America and Europe. Once developed it tends to persist for the rest of the subject's life. It is characterized by 'sleep attacks' or attacks of irresistible sleep lasting on average 10–20 minutes. They commonly occur after eating or while engaged in monotonous tasks but since this is a normal time for sleepiness, the more characteristic feature is the attack occurring under unusual or bizarre circumstances. Thus a patient may describe falling asleep in the middle of being interviewed for a job, dining with others, or during sexual intercourse. The patient awakes refreshed from even brief periods of sleep, and his vigilance is thereby restored for as long as 2 or 3 hours.

In about two-thirds of instances episodes of loss of muscle tone and paralysis also occur, usually triggered by sudden stimuli or emotion such as fear, anger, or laughter (cataplexy). The jaw sags, the eyelids droop and the patient falls with no loss of consciousness. The loss of muscle tone lasts from a few seconds to a few minutes. It may be partial and subtle with loss of tone in the arms reported as clumsiness, or a simple buckling at the knees. In about a third hypnogogic or hypnopompic hallucinations occur just on waking or on going off to sleep. They consist of visual imagery with luminous lights, figures, or complex scenes. Rarest of the accompanying phenomena are episodes of sleep paralysis (about 1 in 4). Again at the transition between sleep and wakefulness the patient finds he cannot move his limbs and is unable to speak. Breathing is unaffected though it may be impossible to take a voluntary deep breath and the eyes may refuse to open. It may take an external trigger to 'break the spell' and allow limb movement. Patients with narcolepsy also describe disturbed nocturnal sleep and automatic behaviour during the day similar to an epileptic fugue.

The narcolepsy syndrome has the strongest association with HLS genotype, 98–99% being DR2 and/or DQw1 positive, an association with the short arm of the 6th chromosome.

Narcolepsy is easy to diagnose when accompanied by cataplexy and sleep paralysis, but the differential diagnosis may have to include epilepsy with fugues, vertebrobasilar ischaemia with cataplectic-like drop attacks. Although the diagnosis is essentially clinical with HLA typing confirmatory, EEG recordings of sleep onset can be helpful. Whilst normals go through stages of increasingly slow wave sleep for some 90 minutes after going to sleep (before entering rapid eye movement 'dreaming' sleep) the narcoleptic patient has REM stages within 10 minutes of at least some sleep onsets. Repeated EEG recordings of sleep onset may be needed to confirm this but much early intrusion of REM sleep is very suggestive of narcolepsy.

Cataplexy responds to drugs like anafranil or may disappear spontaneously. Narcolepsy is a legitimate reason for the regular prescription of amphetamines.

Sleep apnoea syndrome

In this case daytime drowsiness is not as paroxysmal or related to bizarre circumstances and is due to sleep deprivation. This in turn is due to frequent arousals disturbing nocturnal sleep. Collapse of the oropharynx during inspiration causes frequent snoring, choking, gagging and snorting in sleep with partial awakening. The patient is often amnesic about these symptoms (although they may have nightmares, nocturia, and even enuresis) but they are well noted by any partner, who may also be alarmed by obvious pauses in respiration and restlessness bordering on violence. Patients with sleep apnoea are difficult to sleep alongside! The patient may wake with headache and complaining of tiredness and poor concentration as well as of drowsiness. Complaints of memory difficulties, irritability and reduced libido or impotence are common. Driving accidents are likely. Hypertension, polycythaemia, and even cor pulmonale and stroke are serious medical complications.

The usual patient is an overweight middle-aged male with a thick neck (collar size 17" or more), but treatable obstructive airway problems may be obvious on ENT examination (polyps, large tonsils, mandibular deformity). Hypothyroidism and acromegaly can be responsible. Alcohol consumption especially at bedtime is a potent aggravating factor. Positive pressure respiratory support elevating intranasal pressures prevents collapse of the upper airway and allows normal nocturnal sleep, revolutionizing the patient's life.

Hypersomnolence due to hypoventilation in the night may also be seen with dystrophia, myotonica and the muscle weakness of acid maltase deficiency or myasthenia.

Further reading

FISCH, B.J. (1995) Neurological aspects of sleep. In *Neurology and General Medicine*, 2nd edn (ed. M.J. Aminoff), Churchill Livingstone, New York, pp. 491–519.

Memory loss

Complaints of memory impairment are quite common. Often when they come from the patient they prove ill founded; if from a relative they are more often verifiable. This is because poor concentration and lapses of memory are common complaints in depression, anxiety states and in patients distracted by pain or other pressing symptoms. The problem of refuting a patient's insistence that his memory is poor when all other symptoms point to an anxiety state lies in their response to overt memory tests. These are likely to be failed to reinforce the patient's claim. The wealth of detail in the history and the maintenance of work standards may be the best evidence of the lack of organic deficit. Some items of the neuropsychological battery may be useful. Tasks such as picture completion, when the subject is shown rudimentary pictures, or the ability to identify objects photographed from an unusual angle may be 'accidentally' resubmitted, and the improved performance establishes an intact short-term memory. The history of the loss of names for objects may be a sign of dysphasia rather than memory loss, and brief episodes of loss of recall may prove epileptic. A history of loss of memory of personal events and meetings is more likely to be indicative of a dementia.

It is worth noting that psychologists and neurologists tend to use different terms. To the neurologist short-term memory is the ability to recall a name and address over 3 minutes, whilst long-term memory recalls events from childhood. To the psychologist 'short-term memory' refers to immediate recall, e.g. repetition of a string of digits, and all else is long term.

Organic defects of memory are seen with disease of the hippocampi and medial thalamic regions. Temporary amnesia for the content of an attack of temporal lobe epilepsy is usual and helpful in distinguishing it from some other cause of odd behaviour of psychogenic origin. The patient who recalls every word of an argument in an outburst of rage is unlikely to be suffering from temporal lobe epilepsy. The persistence of such mental states for several hours is also unlikely from temporal lobe epilepsy. Amnesia and confusion for some hours may occur, however, with hypoglycaemia and is typical of transient global amnesia (TGA). The patient affected by TGA knows his identity and that of close friends or spouse but constantly asks what they should be doing next. Motor skills are unimpaired. They may have a loss of memory for some days prior to the onset of the attack (retrograde amnesia, RA). This disappears on recovery, leaving only a dense memory loss for the duration of the attack. Most such episodes are single and may be related to migraine. They do not indicate an impending stroke and few are epileptic in nature. Some have been related to sudden immersion in cold water.

Head injury commonly produces a memory gap and the severity of RA and of post-traumatic amnesia (PTA), that interval between recovery of consciousness and of continued recall, are useful measures of the severity of head injury. The duration of PTA exceeds that of RA and one should be suspicious of a complaint of prolonged RA if the PTA is short.

Protracted memory loss with a long RA and ongoing difficulties with registration of new memories may occur after encephalitis affecting the limbic areas (e.g. herpes encephalitis) and after infarction of the hippocampi, e.g. after a basilar artery embolism. Some patients in the early days of temporal lobectomy for epilepsy were left in a similar state if they had a diseased contralateral temporal lobe. Tuberculous meningitis, subarachnoid haemorrhage and carbon monoxide poisoning can all result in comparable deficits. A more slowly evolving difficulty rarely develops with tumours of the floor of the third ventricle. The patients with hippocampal damage may not recall events from a few minutes previously and may fail to recognize their ward attendants, who they see repeatedly each day.

Alcoholic subjects are vulnerable to a particular kind of medial thalamic damage which causes a striking short-term memory defect accompanied in the acute stages by confabulation and disturbed mood (Korsakov's psychosis). Immediate recall of a string of digits is spared but there is profound short-term memory impairment. The amnesia is often accompanied by ataxia, nystagmus and paresis of eye movements due to thiamine deficiency (Wernicke's encephalopathy). The memory defect may prove permanent, whilst the eye signs are usually reversible after an injection of thiamine.

In practice, most patients referred with failing memory will prove to be demented. The history will include evidence from work or family that the patient's ability to cope with everyday intellectual challenges is failing, interest in hobbies flagging and personality changing either to a socially embarrassing disinhibited state or to quiet apathy. Often a crisis, e.g. a bereavement, brings to light a difficulty in coping that had been covered by the now absent spouse, or difficulties at work fail to respond to a holiday and a visit to the general practitioner for a check-up. The patient may have little insight into these changes and may come reluctantly to the consultation to humour his relatives. During the history-taking it may be clear that the patient's memory is poor and that the relative has to provide many of the simple chronological details.

His conversation lacks detail and he fails to expand on the answers to questions. The relative often has to interrupt to fill out the answers or correct errors. The history the patient gives is both brief and at variance with that in the referral letter or from the family. These clues to the presence of dementia are easier to spot than Korsakov's psychosis where confabulation provides rich detail, the errors in which may be unknown to the physician. The dementing patient will show defects of memory and learning in both the verbal and visuospatial areas, e.g. learning of a sentence such as 'The one thing a nation needs to be rich and great is a good secure supply of wood' (Babcock sentence) or a name and address, and the reproduction after brief display of geometric designs (Binet figures). General knowledge will be poor with the patient unaware of recent world events or sporting news even if he declares an interest, unable to name the capital cities of major countries, the names of world leaders or past prime ministers, etc. Difficulties with speech (dysphasia), calculation (dyscalculia) and with visuospatial memory (getting lost in familiar surroundings) may be detectable. Asked to interpret a picture, e.g. an advertisement from a magazine, the patient will often name discrete components of the picture without making the synthesis and 'seeing' that it is an advertisement with a commercial purpose.

It should be stressed that most bedside testing is based on verbal replies and may, therefore, only reflect the performance of the dominant left hemisphere. It is important to test the competence of the minor hemisphere by testing visual learning and memory. In addition to testing the ability to reproduce an abstract figure, it is prudent to check the recognition of famous faces from a newspaper or magazine and perhaps request a drawing or a map of the patient's living room. Any suggestion of sparing of these functions will raise suspicions of a focal dominant hemisphere lesion and prompt formal psychometric confirmation of the restricted nature of the deficit.

Two major groups of conditions cause dementia. Those like Alzheimer's disease are felt to reflect cortical disease, whilst those due to Huntington's chorea, Parkinson's disease and communicating hydrocephalus cause dementia because of sub-cortical damage. Cortical dementia is characterized by aphasia, apraxia, acalculia, and may affect cortical sensory discrimination (astereognosis, graphasthesia). By contrast, sub-cortical dementia shows more striking slowing and personality change without aphasia, etc.

When a memory disorder is accompanied by bedside evidence of dementia, formal psychometry may not be necessary. When changes are not clear cut, or are complicated by depression or dysphasia, then the expertise of a clinical psychologist is needed. The distinction from delirium is important as delirium is usually due to an acute potentially reversible process. It is characterized by over activity, fluctuation, hallucinations and reduced awareness, and there may be a clear history of a sudden onset.

Some 50% of patients whose personality changes or learning and memory defect proves to be due to dementia will prove to have Alzheimer's disease with simple atrophy on CT scanning or MRI. In a small number the aetiology will be suggested by the history. In other cases (Figure 2.7) neuroimaging and blood tests are revealing.

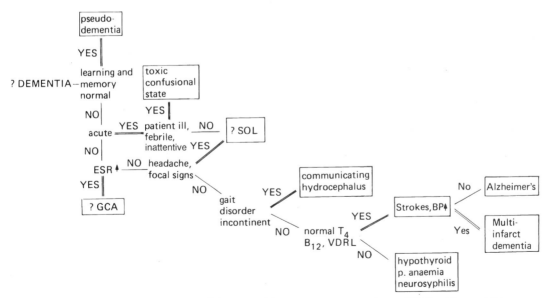

Figure 2.7 Flow chart showing diagnosis of dementia. SOL = space-occupying lesion; VDRL = Venereal Disease Reference Laboratory; GCA = giant cell arteritis.

A family history of dementia suggests Alzheimer's disease or Huntington's chorea, the report of involuntary movements flitting from place to place in chaotic sequence making the latter diagnosis. Dementia may precede chorea by 1–2 years and families may be reluctant to mention a relative who died after years in a mental hospital. Dementia with extrapyramidal features like Parkinsonism, rigidity, or involuntary movements should suggest Parkinson's disease, Creutzfeld–Jakob disease, hydrocephalus, multi-system atrophy, or corticobasal degeneration. The last-named is a rare disorder in which apraxia in a limb is accompanied by rigidity or involuntary movements. The arm may feel foreign and uncontrollable to the patient (alien limb).

A story of sudden onset, stepwise progression with strokes little or large on a background of hypertension or widespread vascular disease, suggests dementia due to multiple areas of cerebral infarction. A 'score' of features culled from the history can suggest the possibility of 'multi-infarct' dementia.

A high alcohol intake suggests alcoholic dementia and other evidence of adverse effects of alcohol on the nervous system such as cerebellar ataxia or a peripheral neuropathy may support the association. The complaint of headache or of focal neurological impairment raises the possibility of a tumour, e.g. frontal meningioma, frontotemporal glioma, corpus callosum glioma, multiple metastases, which must always be sought whether or not there are such clues in the history. This is the major reason to request CT scans or MRI in all demented subjects not found to have neurosyphilis, B_{12} deficiency or hypothyroidism on blood tests.

A scan is also needed to distinguish between the dementia of atrophy (Alzheimer's disease) and that of a communicating hydrocephalus. The history may suggest the latter, with mental slowing associated with the early appearance of incontinence and a difficulty in walking as though the victim had 'forgotten' how to walk. When all three features are present and there is an aetiological explanation for defective cerebrospinal fluid absorption by the arachnoid villi (old meningitis, subarachnoid haemor-

rhage) the dementia will almost certainly improve with the insertion of a ventriculo-venous or ventriculo-peritoneal shunt. The CT scans of such patients show a dilated ventricular system with occluded cortical sulci. By contrast, the scan in a patient suffering from Alzheimer's disease shows combined enlargement of both sulci and ventricles. When the scan is difficult to interpret (e.g. when the sulci over the vertex are occluded but those in the sylvian fissure are prominent), there is no aetiological event and the clinical triad of dementia, gait disorder and incontinence is incomplete, the response to ventricular shunting is unpredictable and often disappointing. As there are risks associated with shunting, especially with the elderly, e.g. 10% get a subdural haematoma, some predictive test would be valuable. Perhaps the best at present consists of the simple clinical observation of the beneficial results of removing 30–60 ml of cerebrospinal fluid by lumbar puncture. Intracranial pressure monitoring may reveal surges of raised intracranial pressure and their presence is predictive of a better outcome from surgery.

Stress is placed on the search for treatable causes of dementia and of conditions masquerading as dementia, since there is currently no effective treatment for Alzheimer's disease. Trials based on the hypothesis that there is defective cholinergic transmission in the cortex have so far met with mixed success. Pseudo-dementia due to depressive slowing and poor concentration is common and it is permissible to embark on a therapeutic trial of antidepressant medication if there is any doubt about the diagnosis. Depression frequently accompanies early dementia so the distinction may need the expertise of psychiatrists and psychologists.

The EEG may help in the distinction, since a normal record (like a normal CT scan or MRI) drives one back upon the history in the attempt to discover whether the patient has an affective disorder. The neurological examination is rarely helpful. Clearly the presence of papilloedema implies that the mental changes are due to a tumour, and the presence of a dyspraxic gait alerts one to a communicating hydrocephalus. Mild lateralizing signs are of low specificity since vascular disease, tumours and simple atrophy may all be accompanied by extensor plantars or even a mild hemiparesis.

The finding of associated parkinsonism raises two possibilities. Firstly, some patients with long-established Parkinson's disease develop intellectual impairment. Secondly, the Steele–Richardson–Olzewski syndrome combines mild dementia with a major defect of vertical eye movement and a mixed picture of rigidity of axial muscles and inco-ordination. The rigidity and an impassive face resemble those in Parkinson's disease, but the brow is more furrowed and the posture less flexed.

Further reading

CUMMINGS, J.L. and BENSON, D.F. (1992) *Dementia: A Clinical Approach*. 2nd edn. Butterworth-Heinemann, London.

VICTOR, M. (1969) The amnesic syndrome and its anatomical basis. *Can. Med. Assoc. J.*, 100, 1115.

WHITTY, C.W.M. and ZANGWILL, O.L. (1984) *Amnesia*, 3rd edn. Butterworths, London.

Visual symptoms

Visual failure

Early diagnosis is vital if sight is to be saved. The tempo of the history, the appearance of the eye and optic nerve and the nature of the field defect are the corner-stones of the bed-side assessment. It should be noted that lesions at the chiasm or in front of it cause a reduction in visual acuity, whilst those in the tract or radiation do not, causing instead a field defect that the patient may not have noticed. Lesions of the cornea, lens and vitre-ous affect acuity but do not cause a field defect or affect the pupillary reflex. Patients may not know whether their loss of vision applies to one eye or to a homonymous field defect. As the temporal half-field is larger, a right-sided hemianopia is often misinterpreted by its vic-tim as loss of vision in the right eye. If the physician is lucky, the patient reporting a tem-porary loss will have covered each eye in turn

and discovered the truth for himself. If not, the only clue can be the insistence that they lost 'half of everything' which implies a hemiano-pia rather than monocular visual loss, as does the story of 'bumping into things on the left'. The distinction is easy if symptoms persist but is difficult when the patient is relating a prior ischaemic attack. The practical point is that monocular attacks imply carotid artery dis-ease, and hemianopic episodes usually imply vertebrobasilar ischaemia.

Acute loss of vision is usually due to a vascu-lar cause with vessel occlusion causing ischae-mia of the retina or visual cortex. When it affects a single eye there is always the possibility that the patient has accidentally and acutely discov-ered a longer-lasting defect, for example by rub-bing the other eye. A careful history of how the visual loss was detected may reveal this state of affairs, when it must be accepted that the loss may or may not have been sudden. Acute ischaemia of the eye may occur briefly (amaurosis fugax) when embolic occlusion of the central retinal artery causes a black-out of the whole uniocular field for 3–4 minutes. As the embolus of cardiac or carotid origin breaks up or moves recovery commences, perhaps relieving ischaemia in one half of the retina before the other. This explains the story given by the patient that their blurring cleared like a shutter from above or below, passing through a stage when they could see the upper or lower half only. Such a horizontal meridian in a pre-scribed field in one eye always implicates the retina or optic nerve and is usually a reflection of vascular disease. Persisting occlusion of the retinal artery causes permanent loss of retinal function with infarction, a blind eye with visible abnormalities of the retinal vessels which look pale and threadlike. Painless acute loss of vision can also be due to a vitreous haemorrhage visible with the ophthalmoscope and by retinal detachment, which the inexperienced can find more difficult to see.

If the optic nerve suffers a similar fate, as in giant cell arteritis, the visual loss is also likely to be permanent. There may in the acute stage be some slight swelling of the optic nerve head due to ischaemic oedema of the optic nerve. The retinal vessels are normal in the acute stage. When acute loss of vision occurs in both eyes from occipital ischaemia, there is no visible abnormality of the retina or optic nerve, of course, and pupillary reflexes are normal. Optokinetic nystagmus, observed whilst the patient concentrates on the stripes on a rotating drum or the figures on a tape measure passed across his gaze, is lost. Temporary bilateral blurring may occur during transient embolic ischaemia in the basilar artery or in migraine when positive phenomena are likely. Thus the patient describes flashing lights, zigzag lines and shapes like the battlements of castles expanding to fill the visual field, usually in advance of the nauseating headache. Such episodes rarely exceed 30 minutes. With infarction of the occipital cortex producing blindness there may be associated denial of blindness (Anton's syndrome) with patients describing scenes when facing a blank wall.

Subacute loss of vision in one eye is commonly due to optic neuritis (retrobulbar neuritis) which in turn is commonly associated with the eventual appearance of other manifestations of multiple sclerosis (rarer causes include sarcoidosis). The patient describes the rapid blurring of vision in one eye over a few days, with loss of colour appreciation and the appearance of a central area of maximal loss (central scotoma). There is often some aching in the eye when it is moved, due to traction on the optic nerve undergoing demyelination. On examination acuity is reduced, colour vision lost, the pupillary response is sluggish to direct stimulation and there is a central scotoma. Initially the disc looks normal or slightly swollen. Pallor develops rapidly in many. Over the course of some 6 weeks most get excellent recovery of vision. Residual difficulties may be experienced with colour, and the swinging light test may reveal a relative afferent pupillary defect (see p. 23). Acuity may fall after a hot bath or in hot weather. Visual evoked potentials disappear when acuity falls and on recovery may be prolonged: a useful marker of a past episode of optic neuritis. Retinal causes for loss of acuity can usually be distinguished from those arising in the optic nerve from the fundoscopic appearances. Micropsia and distortion of visual images also suggest retinal disease, e.g. oedema at the macula, whilst striking colour vision loss points more to an optic nerve lesion. Other causes of central field loss (besides optic nerve disease) include macula disease and scotomatous bitemporal defects from a lesion at the back of the chiasm where the fibres from the maculae decussate. They can be vulnerable if a pituitary tumour develops in a patient whose chiasm is anteriorly sited (pre-fixed chiasm). Careful field testing detects the bitemporal nature of the central defects. Central scotomas also occur with the visual loss of B_{12} deficiency and tobacco amblyopia. These scotomata lie between the blindspot and fixation, and are most obvious using a red test object.

If recovery of visual acuity is not occurring in an apparent optic neuritis or there is any evidence of progression (visual acuity falling further, scotoma enlarging, field of other eye becoming affected), then the rival possibility of compression of the optic nerve or chiasm must be pursued energetically. High resolution CT scanning or MRI of the orbit and chiasmatic region is the procedure of first choice. Exploration is now rarely needed but should still be considered if visual failure progresses without a diagnosis being made.

Rarely, progressive loss is due to multiple sclerosis but this diagnosis is only possible if the other features of the disease are clear cut. B_{12} deficiency or the toxic effects of tobacco in pipe smokers can cause a progressive visual impairment with bilateral scotomas to a small red object between the fixation point and the blind spot. This change is reversible if the patient is given vitamins including hydroxycobalamine. Tobacco amblyopia is rare now and was mostly seen with a combination of heavy drinking and pipe smoking. Rarely, a hereditary optic neuropathy can cause slowly progressive loss, often levelling out short of complete blindness.

Hysterical visual loss is suspected when pupillary responses are normal, optokinetic nystagmus easily detected and the patient avoids self-injury in an unfamiliar room.

Double vision

If the defective eye movement is not obvious on immediate inspection of conjugate gaze to the left, right, up and down, attention to the behaviour of images will often reveal the culprit. Diplopia only at a distance implies a 6th nerve palsy and diplopia only for near objects suggests a difficulty in accommodation, rarely of neurological significance. Horizontal separation of images suggests weakness of a horizontal movement. Vertical diplopia implies weakness of a vertically acting muscle. Oblique separation of images usually results from weakness of a vertically acting muscle. If vertical or oblique diplopia can be corrected by head tilt a 4th nerve palsy is suspected. Tilting the head to the side of a 4th nerve lesion increases separation of the images; tilting away from the side of the lesion obliterates the diplopia. A slight turn of the head may be a sign of compensation for a lateral separation of images as due to a 6th nerve palsy.

The patient is next asked to say when, in the course of following the examiner's finger, maximum separation occurs. It is in fact best to use a finer target at this stage, e.g. a pencil or an orange stick. The outer or more peripheral image is then due to the weak eye and this can be simply determined by closing or obstructing the view of each of the patient's eyes in turn and requesting that he reports which image (the nearer or the further out) disappears. The weak muscle or movement is that which the weak eye was doing when the doubling occurred. Attention can then be directed to whether an individual nerve palsy is responsible or if the disorder of the eye movement is more complex. A 3rd nerve palsy causes diplopia in all directions except when that eye is abducted, and there will usually be a telltale ptosis. A 4th nerve palsy causes vertical diplopia with maximum separation of images on down gaze to the side that requires adduction of the affected eye. The 6th nerve palsy is easiest of all, with progressive horizontal separation as abduction increases.

More complex eye movement derangement producing diplopia may be caused by thyroid disease, when proptosis and lid retraction are usual, and by myasthenia, when there is fatiguable ptosis, normal pupil size and a positive response to edrophonium. As the patient refixes on the level after looking downwards the upper lid may overshoot, momentarily baring the sclera. This eyelid twitch was noted by Cogan to be a sign of myasthenia. Thyroid disease is often responsible if only one of the muscles innervated by the 3rd nerve is affected. Ptosis and immobility of the eyes may be seen with ocular myopathy (no diplopia) and with supranuclear ophthalmoplegias in which movement to head rotation still occurs. Diplopia or polyopia (multiple images) in one eye can be hysterical but is often due to local disease of the eye such as a dislocated lens, posterior polar cataracts, keratoconus or retinal detachment. Often, however, the patient means that the vision in that eye is blurred due to reduced acuity and not that there are two or more images. A patient may report triple vision with one image from the good eye and two from the other. Multiple images (polyopia) can be caused by occipital lesions.

Some other visual symptoms

Photophobia, the avoidance of bright light, occurs with meningeal irritation whether from blood (subarachnoid haemorrhage) or from infection (meningitis). It is also complained of in inflammation of the eye (conjunctivitis) and in any condition that causes a dilated pupil and may be present during convalescence from a field defect of vascular origin in the hemisphere. It also occurs in migraine.

Visual hallucinations arise from the occipital lobe (coloured shapes or blobs) or from the temporal lobe (complex scenes) or cerebral peduncle (geometric patterns). Flashes or sparks may arise from disease of the retina or optic nerve.

Oscillopsia or movement of the visual world develops with nystagmus, especially of peripheral labyrinthine origin. Bouncing of the visual world when walking is experienced with bilateral labyrinthine damage as caused by ototoxic drugs, e.g. gentamycin. It is also mentioned by patients with downbeat nystagmus due to a lesion at the foramen magnum, or cerebellar degeneration.

Haloes around objects, as when a street light is viewed through the rain, are reported by patients with glaucoma and also accompany cataracts and some corneal diseases.

Head tilt is usually due to weakness of the superior oblique muscle with vertical separation and oblique displacement of images. The head is tilted away from the affected eye. It is also seen with spasm of sub-occipital muscles on one side which may be a sign of a cerebellar tumour. Combined with rotation of the neck, it forms part of the movement disorder, torticollis. The posture may be maintained tonically or be accompanied by irregular jerks.

Metamorphopsia, a complaint that images are small, large or distorted, is usually a sign of retinal disease, usually of the macula.

Night blindness reflects failure of rod function in the peripheral retina and is often accompanied by restriction of the peripheral field. The most important cause is retinitis pigmentosa, identified ophthalmoscopically by peripherally placed pigment often looking like little spiders or bone corpuscles. The electroretinogram is useful in early diagnosis. A very restricted field is also seen in advanced glaucoma, and sometimes evinced by a hysterical patient. The field may then be as small at the back of the room as close-to, or spiral in on repeated testing.

Facial pain

Here is another situation, like the problem of headache, in which little help can be expected from the examination, and details of the history are crucial.

Acute attacks

The appearance for a day or two of facial pain over the forehead or cheek may be due to acute sinusitis. This pain may vary with posture, be aggravated or relieved by blowing the nose and accompanied by a blocked nose or nasal discharge. The patient may be febrile and the area over the affected sinus tender.

Sinusitis is rare without nasal symptoms. Tooth-ache is a dull boring pain that may throb. It is likely to be affected by the temperature of food or drink, and can be provoked by percussing the responsible tooth. A burning pain, over the forehead on one side for example, may be the harbinger of the diagnostic vesicles of herpes zoster infection. A similar pain spreading to the back of the head with associated claudication of the jaw during chewing, scalp tenderness, and constitutional symptoms is indicative of giant cell arteritis. There may be exquisite tenderness, redness, beading, and loss of pulsation in the superficial temporal arteries, but they may also be normal.

Shooting pains

These are diagnostic of trigeminal neuralgia and usually affect the angle of the mouth. Severe stabs of pain occur in runs with only a mild background pain. The individual stabs, which last only seconds, may be triggered by touching the face, chewing, cold air, cleaning teeth or talking. The wince with each pain gives rise to the name 'tic douloureux'. The patient, if symptomatic, will commonly give his history with a minimum of facial movement, hardly moving his lips after the style of a ventriloquist. He will point to the site of the pain without letting the finger touch the skin. An animated verbose description of facial pain with much rubbing of the face is most unlikely to be due to trigeminal neuralgia. Carbamazepine, baclofen, clonazepam or surgical attack on the 5th nerve are the mainstays of treatment. Thermocoagulation of the nerve is the first-choice procedure for most surgeons, but some prefer to explore the nerve root in younger patients in case it shows signs of compression by an aberrant vessel, which can be relieved.

Periodic pain

Migraine may affect the face, producing a throbbing pain around the eye and cheek for half a day at a time. The patient will usually describe periodic headaches as well.

Migrainous neuralgia affects the middle-aged and causes attacks of severe pain lasting 30–45 minutes at a time (Figure 2.8). They may recur daily for many weeks and then abate for, say, 18 months before returning in another cluster. Attacks may wake the patient in a bizarre regular fashion, e.g. at 2.15 each morning. Some patients develop a small pupil on the side of the pain. The only migrainous thing is their response to ergotamine, sumatryptan, and methysergide. Oxygen may abort an individual pain and lithium carbonate is currently the best prophylactic regimen for chronic sufferers. Women with the chronic syndrome may respond to indomethacin.

Continuous pain

Occasionally nasopharyngeal tumours may present with facial pain, and all such patients should have an ENT examination of the posterior nasopharyngeal space. Much more commonly, no such lesion will be found and the patient's facial pain appears to be the equivalent of a tension headache. Many of the victims are depressed middle-aged women who rub their faces as they describe the day-in, day-out pain. They have usually had extensive

dental extractions, correction of their bite to take stress off the temporomandibular joint, correction of minor refraction errors and sinus wash-outs or drainage procedures. The history after such intervention may be 'lost in antiquity'. A trial of antidepressants is the next best move.

Vertigo

It is helpful to consider the vestibular system as two balanced halves with tonic activity in the vestibular end organs, brain stem and neck reflexes. Normal head movement causes an imbalance of such activity with a perception of movement and corrective ocular deviation. If disease of the end organ or brain stem leads to imbalance, there is illusory movement (vertigo) and inappropriate eye movement (nystagmus). Clinically, true vertigo, which involves an hallucination of movement, needs to be distinguished from the light-headedness of anxiety and syncope. Once it is decided that a feeling of swaying, pitching or rotation is being described, the problem becomes that of deciding whether the lesion is in the peripheral labyrinth and 8th nerve or in the brain stem. The distinction can usually be made at the bedside, with careful assessment of nystagmus **(pp 29-30)**. The vertigo (see Table 1.8, p. 30) of a peripheral disturbance is short-lived (only 3 weeks) and often accompanied by a severe systemic disturbance. There is associated unidirectional horizontal nystagmus that is of greatest amplitude when gaze is in the direction of the fast component (Alexander's law). There is no vertical nystagmus. The horizontal nystagmus is enhanced or brought out by loss of ocular fixation which can be conveniently checked by the use of Frenzel's glasses, whose high plus lenses prevent focusing while allowing the examiner a magnified view of the patient's eyes. It may be possible to achieve the same result by getting the patient to close one eye while the movement is observed at the retina

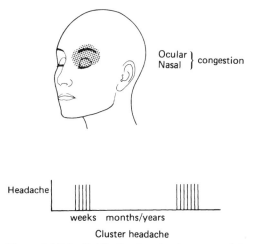

Figure 2.8 Pain distribution in migrainous neuralgia.

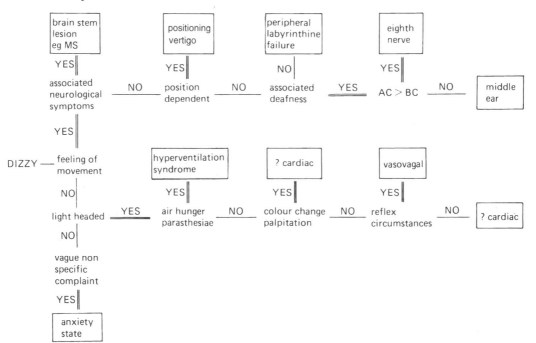

Figure 2.9 Flow chart in the diagnosis of vertigo.

with an ophthalmoscope which obscures the view of the second eye.

The nystagmus that accompanies vertigo of brain-stem origin is usually multidirectional, can be vertical and outlasts any symptoms of vertigo. It may persist for years. Systemic symptoms are less prominent and the nystagmus is not enhanced by loss of fixation. Nystagmus in a non-vertiginous subject can be assumed to be central in origin.

Most 'peripheral' causes of vertigo are due to acute labyrinthine failure. In young people this is often attributed to acute labyrinthitis but an infective cause has not been proved. After a few days of spontaneous vertigo, the dizzy sensation and nystagmus subside together. The nausea, vomiting, pallor and sweating that accompany the onset of vertigo may occasion a mistaken diagnosis of myocardial infarction until the unwilling eyelids are prised open to reveal the severe nystagmus. Similar vertigo occurring in late life is usually attributed to a vascular cause. Occlusion of the vestibular branch of the internal auditory artery is assumed but

proof is lacking. Episodes of peripheral labyrinthine dysfunction also occur in Ménière's disease with increased endolymphatic pressure. Tinnitus and hearing loss with loudness recruitment accompany the vertigo, and a sense of fullness in the ear may precede attacks. Rupture of the round window after head injury or barotrauma and spread of infection from otitis media require urgent ENT referral if they are suspected.

Central causes of vertigo include multiple sclerosis in younger subjects and vascular disease in older people. The brain-stem origin of symptoms is confirmed by accompanying complaints of diplopia, facial sensory disturbance, dysarthria, etc. and the time course of events confirms the pathological diagnosis. Little vertigo is described by patients with tumours in the cerebellopontine angle who have deafness, with or without loss of corneal reflex at the time of presentation.

Ototoxic drugs like streptomycin and gentamicin cause no vertigo but they produce bilateral labyrinthine damage as revealed by loss of caloric responsiveness and loss of balance. The victims are left highly dependent on visual clues and have great difficulty with balance in poor lighting. This can be revealed by getting them to walk on an unpredictable surface such as a mattress, with their eyes closed. As they walk in the street their visual world may bob up and down (oscillopsia).

Vertigo related to change of posture, e.g. when bending over, reaching up, lying down and sitting up, is called positioning vertigo and is usually associated with benign positioning nystagmus. It is seen after head injury and after acute labyrinthine failure, but may develop in isolation. Simple advice on avoiding the rapid provocative movements may be all that is needed as the prognosis is good, though recently introduced particle repositioning procedures like those described by Semont and Epley are said to be successful in 80% of instances. Minor head injuries are often followed by complaints of headache, poor concentration and memory, and of dizziness. Whilst the post-concussion syndrome is sometimes psychogenically elaborated, especially when the head injury is subject to litigation, it is important to realise that all of these may be organic sequelae. Migraine can be triggered in susceptible individuals and the dizziness often proves to be of the type seen with damage to the labyrinth (benign positioning vertigo).

The duration of vertigo may be helpful in the differential diagnosis. That due to benign positioning vertigo lasts seconds only; that in Ménière's disease usually lasts for hours whilst the vertigo of vestibular 'neuronitis' continues for a few days, petering out over 2 or 3 weeks. Momentary dizziness is usually due to anxiety.

If the patient also complains of deafness its time course is also important. A sudden onset of deafness and vertigo implies an infectious or vascular cause, whilst episodic fluctuating deafness suggests Ménière's disease. A slowly progressive deafness should raise suspicions of an acoustic neuroma.

Associated symptoms may lead one to suspect a brain-stem lesion (facial numbness, slurred speech and poor co-ordination) an aural cause (deafness and tinnitus) or hyperventilation (paraesthesiae, tightness in the chest, a lump in the throat).

Loss of balance

Unsteadiness without a subjective sense of dizziness or vertigo may be due to bilateral labyrinthine damage, cerebellar dysfunction, or loss of position sense. It is aggravated by poor vision and leg weakness, and is often multifactorial in origin, especially in the elderly, who complain of unsteadiness and falls. Impaired postural reflexes and adjustments also cause falls in patients with Parkinson's disease.

The examination thus concentrates on a search for cerebellar deficit or sensory loss. Cerebellar signs may be restricted to ataxia of gait and stance with perhaps some ataxia of the legs but little of the arms, and perhaps with no dysarthria or nystagmus: the picture of midline or diffuse cerebellar lesions.

A slowly-evolving picture in a young person suggests a hereditary cause such as Friedreich's ataxia, in which scoliosis and pes cavus are common and absent ankle jerks are combined with extensor plantar responses although ataxia is the dominant cause of disability. In middle life a progressive ataxia may be accompanied by dementia, eye movement disorders, optic atrophy and retinal pigmentation. In the elderly, dementia may be the only accompanying sign. Alcohol, antiepileptic drugs and lithium may cause a toxic cerebellar ataxia. Metabolic problems that have the same effect include hypothyroidism, vitamin E deficiency and Wilson's disease. A cerebellar deficit may complicate infections such as chicken pox, mumps, rubella, infectious mononucleosis, brucella, Creutzfeld–Jakob disease and Whipple's disease. Ataxia may appear as a paraneoplastic complication of a systemic malignancy.

Joint position sense loss is detected by testing the awareness of small movements of the toes, and by a positive Romberg's sign. It may be revealing to have the patient shoot at his big toe with his index finger while his eyes are shut, whilst the examiner moves the target about above the bed with different degrees of flexion of the hip, knee and ankle. In those with sensory ataxia faulty tracking with the

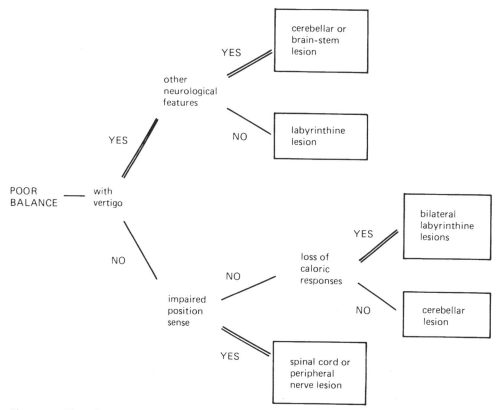

Figure 2.10 Flow chart in the diagnosis of the cause of poor balance.

finger is striking. Causes include peripheral neuropathies and spinal cord disease, such as tabes dorsalis. Bilateral labyrinthine disease is suspected on the basis of a history of ototoxic medication, and the discovery of absent caloric responses.

Further reading

BRANDT, D. (1991) *Vertigo — its Multisensory Syndromes.* Springer Verlag, London.

BALOH, R.W. and HONRUBIA, V. (1990) *Clinical Neurophysiology of the Vestibular System.* F.A. Davis, Philadelphia.

Dysarthria

Speech production needs the co-ordination of respiration, laryngeal and supralaryngeal movements. Poor diction or articulation gives rise to defective pronunciation of words, though the language content of the speech is unimpaired, thus distinguishing the problem from dysphasia. If the patient's speech, however difficult to 'catch', is transcribed or the patient writes the same message, the grammar is normal and the words are all correct. Only their sound is at fault (Table 2.3).

Many neurological problems affect diction. Loss of the lower motor neurones from cranial nerve palsies can affect speech. A flaccid cheek or lip, even on one side from a Bell's palsy,

Table 2.3 Dysarthria

Lesion	Condition	Speech quality
Extrapyramidal	Parkinson's	Monotonous, quiet, mumbling
	Dystonia	Tight, slow
Cerebellar	Multiple sclerosis	Drunken slurring or explosive staccato
Upper motor neurone (bilateral)	Pseudobulbar palsy (motor neurone disease or bilateral strokes)	Spastic – sounds like pebble in mouth
Lower motor neurone (bilateral)	Motor neurone disease	Nasal with poor definition

produces an altered sound quality which can be mimicked by holding one's cheek back with a finger in the corner of the mouth. B,P,M,W are difficult to say without movement of the lips as any ventriloquist would confess. Bilateral loss of bulbar function, e.g. from motor neurone disease or bulbar polio, also makes P's and B's very soft and, in addition it is difficult to repeat V's and I's. The voice has a nasal quality if the palate is paralysed and the nasal escape of air can be heard or seen by placing a cold mirror at the nasal orifice while the patient says 'pa, pa, pa'. The problem is aggravated by flexion of the head. If the tongue is wasted and becoming immobile in the floor of the mouth, clarity is further impaired. T,S, and D are especially difficult without normal tongue control. A voice that starts a telephone conversation or lecture normally but becomes nasal with fatigue indicates myasthenia gravis.

Upper motor neurone lesions cause dysarthria when bilateral. The stiff spastic slowly-moving tongue makes the speech sound as though the individual has a pebble in his mouth. The mouth tends not to be fully opened. The speech may be slightly nasal, S, Z and V are difficult and repetition (pa, pa, pa or la, la, la) slow and laboured. Unilateral lesions cause only transient disturbance of speech and swallowing, though Broca aphasia is sometimes accompanied by dysarthria due to difficulty in carrying out complex motor tasks with mouth and tongue. Such

'dyspraxia' is often revealed by failure to blow a kiss, flick jam off the top lip, etc., even though there is no major paralysis of the muscles involved. Rhythm and stress of syllables are impaired. It can be difficult to distinguish from intonation alone between a phrase used as either a question or an answer.

Parkinson's disease produces a low volume, quiet monotonous mumbling speech that eventually becomes incoherent. The poverty or economy of finger movements seen in carrying out the five finger exercise is matched by lack of full range and fluent movements of tongue and lips. Festination of gait may be matched by acceleration of speech. Pa, pa, pa becomes hummed with deteriorating clarity of the P. Other patients with extrapyramidal disorders have a sound quality mimicked by tightening the muscles of the larynx and pharynx: so-called dystonic speech. The voice sounds rather like that of a dalek.

Cerebellar disease produces either a simple slurring with imprecise consonants, as when drunk, or an interrupted flow, the words being spat out explosively like unpunctuated writing. Loudness fluctuates more than usual and separate syllables get undue stress. Such 'scanning' staccato speech of a monotonous sing-song quality is often heard from patients with disturbance of cerebellar connections due to multiple sclerosis. Words individually take longer to say and vowel sounds particularly are lengthened.

Thus in most situations the examiner can assess the type of lesion responsible for dysarthria simply by listening to the speech. Confirmation comes from the other neurological signs of cerebellar ataxia, parkinsonism, cranial nerve palsies, pseudobulbar palsy, etc.

Further reading

ROSENFIELD, D.B. and BARROSO, A.O. (1991) Dysarthria, dysfluency and dysphagia. In *Neurology and Clinical Practice* Bradley W.C. et al. (eds.). Butterworth-Heinemann, Boston.

ALEXANDER, M.P. and BENSON, D.F. (1991) The aphasias and related disturbances. In *Clinical Neurology*, vol. 1 (ed. R.J. Joynt), JB Lippincott, Philadelphia.

Dysphonia

This includes disturbed vocalization as in laryngitis, but it also occurs in a neurological context, for example with vocal cord paralysis. A defective cough suggests the latter and laryngoscopy is diagnostic.

Hysterical loss of voice is suspected when the cough is normal but phonation is only possible in a whisper, meaning that adduction of the vocal cords occurs reflexly but not voluntarily.

The strength of the voice fades away during conversation in the myasthenic, and the parkinsonian patient has a persistently quiet voice. The sound quality of the voice in dystonia may be 'strangled'.

Hearing loss

This is usually a problem for the ENT specialist but neurologists are sometimes called upon to make the initial assessment.

Sudden loss of hearing on one side may be due to infections such as mumps or herpes zoster. A sudden vascular occlusion may also cause deafness but this is usually accompanied by vertigo as the vestibular nerve is also affected. After head injury or a rapid change of altitude, the round window may rupture producing sudden conductive deafness. Syphilis and multiple sclerosis are also occasional causes.

Progressive loss of hearing which is sensorineural in type is often due to acoustic trauma or to age (presbyacusis). Ménière's disease is also a cause but is complicated by tinnitus and attacks of vertigo. An acoustic neuroma may cause unilateral deafness before it also affects balance. Quinine, ethacrynic acid, frusemide, and aspirin may cause a reversible toxic deafness whilst that due to aminoglycosides may be permanent. Total deafness will usually prove to be perceptive in type. Conductive deafness may be due to otosclerosis or chronic infection of the middle ear. Audiometry and

ENT help will be needed in sorting out all these problems. The aetiological diagnosis will often depend on other features of the case such as evidence of vascular disease or of brain-stem dysfunction.

Tinnitus

Patients may hear the sound of flow in AVMs or in a stenosed carotid artery, that the doctor can also hear. More commonly the complaint of a persistent sound, usually a high pitched whistle, is due to disease of the ear (otosclerosis, Ménière's), or systemic factors such as anaemia, fever or the effect of drugs such as aspirin in high dose. In many patients there is no clear abnormality, despite the distressing symptom.

Further reading

BALLANTYNE, J., MARTIN, M.C. and MARTIN, A.M. (1993) *Deafness*, 5th edn. Churchill Livingstone, Edinburgh.

Pain

Pain arises either from tissue injury with stimulation of the endings of small nerve fibres or from disease of the peripheral nerve or central pathways themselves, up to and including the thalamus.

Peripheral nerve

Mechanical injury to peripheral nerves (as in wartime or with mechanical accidents) can be followed by severe burning pain (causalgia). It is usually accompanied by hypersensitivity, swelling, hyperhidrosis, and eventually trophic skin changes. Osteoporosis of bones may follow, partly due to immobility as the patient protects the affected part, e.g. cradling an injured hand to avoid all contact on its shiny sensitive skin. The median nerve and sciatic nerve are the most often affected. The pain is increased by dependency and emotional stress. The skin becomes thin and cool though sweaty, and may be cyanosed. The pain is relieved by sympathetic block, sympathectomy or regional intravenous guanethidine blocks which may help diagnostically. The same picture accompanied by a frozen shoulder may follow myocardial infarction. Sometimes there is no history of damage to either the peripheral or central nervous systems.

Occasionally the problem is iatrogenic; an ulnar nerve may be transposed to arrest the wasting and weakness of chronic entrapment at the elbow, only to cause persistent burning pain of causalgic type.

Peripheral nerve entrapment may cause pain along with sensory disturbance and weakness. The familiar carpal tunnel syndrome may cause pain in the hand, wrist and arm, especially at night, when it is relieved by hanging the arm out of bed. The patient describes a flicking of the painful hand to gain relief, which is fairly diagnostic. Ulnar nerve entrapment at the elbow can cause an ache in the hypothenar eminence and ulnar border of the forearm, often worse in cold weather. The paraesthesiae in the ulnar two fingers are often painful. Compression of lower limb nerves is less often a source of pain, although the tarsal tunnel syndrome with entrapment of plantar nerves may be a cause of pain in the sole of the foot. Femoral nerve damage, e.g. in diabetes mellitus, may cause pain in the front of the thigh and entrapment of the lateral cutaneous nerve of the thigh in the groin leads to pain, paraesthesiae and numbness on the outer side of the thigh in an area the size of the patient's hand (meralgia paraesthetica).

In all entrapment neuropathies there may be indications for surgical decompression to relieve pain. Femoral neuropathy may respond to diabetic control and meralgia paraesthetica to weight loss, if its development coincided with weight gain, as is often the case.

Peripheral neuropathy occasionally causes pain in the legs (e.g. diabetic, amyloid, HIV and alcoholic neuropathies). The calves may be tender.

Brachial plexus

Distressing pain may develop after brachial plexus damage sustained in a motor-cycle accident. The patient's head and shoulder strike the road, causing traction on the plexus and roots. The resulting flail arm may be the site of distressing persistent pain.

Pain may also develop and be followed by rapid wasting and weakness after viral illnesses or vaccinations (brachial plexitis or neuralgic amyotrophy). The pain usually abates in a few weeks but the wasting and weakness may take many months to improve.

Malignant infiltration of the brachial plexus or damage by radiation may cause pain and progressive neurological deficit in the arm of a patient with carcinoma of the breast. Pain in the hand may be due to carpal tunnel pressure in a lymphoedematous arm but usually the pain originates in the plexus, the patient showing diffuse weakness and loss of tendon reflexes in that arm. If a mass can be felt the usual cause is an infiltration and radiation may be helpful. If there is no palpable mass and the patient has already had axillary irradiation, the distinction between infiltration and radiation fibrosis may be impossible without surgical exploration, though the lower plexus is more often involved in infiltration with sparing of the shoulder. MRI may be able to make the distinction. If the prognosis is bad because of metastatic disease, or in the case of an inoperable Pancoast's tumour affecting the lower cord of the plexus, a spinothalamic tractotomy can give pain relief for some 6 months. This is not a good choice if the patient has several years of life ahead of him, since the pain control, although good, is only temporary.

Dorsal root ganglia

These are invaded and damaged by the herpes zoster virus, giving rise to pain of root distribution prior to the eruption of the telltale vesicles. Later post-herpetic neuralgia may develop. This distressing pain, which is particularly likely to follow herpes zoster infection in the elderly, may slowly fade over the years but is difficult to treat. Local ice, cold sprays and vibrators on the edge of the painful area may all help, as may combinations of amitriptyline with carbamazepine or sodium valproate. Transcutaneous nerve stimulation is only rarely helpful and pain pathway surgery often contraindicated by the patient's frail elderly state. Occasionally additional, very brief lancinating pains occur and these may respond to carbamazepine.

Lancinating pains are more frequently encountered in the damage done to the dorsal root ganglia in tabes dorsalis due to syphilis. Tabes dorsalis may be delayed 20–30 years after primary infection. The brunt of the damage falls on the central processes of dorsal root ganglion cells with secondary degeneration of the dorsal columns, hence tabes *dorsalis*. Patients develop ataxia, worse in the dark, classically falling when bending over a wash bowl and closing their eyes when washing their faces. Ankle jerks are usually lost and vibration sense and joint position sense impaired. Lightning pains like knives piercing the lower leg at right angles are common, along with paraesthesiae. Odd patches of sensory loss may be found over the nose, sternum, inner aspect of the forearm and outer side of the lower leg. The bladder is often affected and becomes atonic and distended with overflow incontinence. With loss of deep pain sensation in the legs, there being no discomfort on Achilles tendon pressure, destructive but painless arthritis of the knee or ankle joint may develop, a 'Charcot' joint.

Nerve root

Nerve root pain is commonly due to degenerative disease of the cervical or lumbar spine. It tends to be described by the patient with terms like stinging, burning, searing, and sharp. Lumbar disc prolapse characteristically causes root pain (sciatica) increased by sitting, coughing and sneezing, and relieved by lying

flat or even by walking. Straight leg raising is painful, and the pain is exacerbated by trying to put the chin on the chest, as this also stretches the now tethered root. Osteoarthritis of the lumbar spine can also cause root pain without disc prolapse, especially when there is congenital narrowing of the canal, predisposing the patient to compression of roots in the extended posture. In this the pain develops during standing and walking but can be relieved by sitting. Straight leg raising often has no aggravating effect on the pain. These patients find that they can get some relief by walking with a slight stoop, and cycling is less painful as it maintains a flexed lower spine. The pain tends to take 5–10 minutes to abate if they stop walking. By contrast, exercise pain in the leg due to ischaemia of muscles is relieved much quicker and is associated with loss of peripheral pulses and no neurological deficit. To be sure of the distinction these patients must be examined after symptomatic exercise to see whether they lose pulses or develop root signs. In the upper limb root pain may relate to neck movement, but coughing and sneezing are less often provocative.

Root pain may not only be referred to the dermatome supplied by the sensory root. In addition pain may be felt in the muscles (myotome). The distribution of pain commonly encountered with the most frequently affected roots is as follows:

1. *C6 root (C5/6 disc)*. Pain is often felt at the ridge of the trapezius, at the shoulder, in the biceps and over the radial side of the forearm with paraesthesiae in the thumb and index.
2. *C7 root (C6/7 disc)*. Here pain is appreciated over the shoulder blade, in the pectoral region, over the posterolateral aspect of the upper arm and on the back of the forearm with paraesthesiae in the middle finger.
3. *L4 root (L3/4 disc)*. Pain is located in the anterior aspect of the thigh and at the medial side of the knee. Passive extension of the hip stretching the femoral nerve may be limited by pain (positive femoral stretch test). Any paraesthesiae may extend below the knee on the medial side.

4. *L5 root (L4/5 disc)*. Pain radiates down the outer side of the leg into the region of the tibialis anterior with paraesthesiae on the lateral aspect of the lower leg and on the top of the foot.
5. *S1 root (L5/s1 disc)*. The pain is felt in the back of the thigh·and in the side of the foot where any paraesthesiae are felt. With both L5 and S1 root entrapment, straight leg raising may be restricted and painful. It is worth noting that elevation of the other leg may also be restricted as it causes flexion of the spine, which may be painful or may increase contralateral sciatica. It is advisable to check that elevation of the flexed leg is not also painful, since this is a sign of hip joint disease, not of root irritation. External and internal rotation of the hip, with the knee flexed, test whether hip movement is free and pain free.

In cranial nerves irritation of the most proximal part of the nerve intracranially may cause lancinating pains reminiscent of those provoked by lesions of dorsal root ganglia. Severe but very brief pains strike in the territory of the trigeminal or glossopharyngeal nerves (and occasionally in the occipital nerve). Exploration of the intracranial portion of the nerve may reveal a vascular anomaly or small vessel in contact with the root. Separation of the structures relieves the pain but this is a major procedure and should be avoided in the elderly. Antiepileptic drugs are usually effective, e.g. carbamazepine.

If the glossopharyngeal nerve is affected, pain is felt in the tonsillar bed and ear and is triggered by swallowing. The same drugs can be tried and if necessary the nerve is sectioned or its root explored.

Spinal cord

Damage to the pain pathways ascending in the spinal cord can cause a burning pain and hypersensitivity below the level of the lesion. The commonest cause for such a lesion is probably multiple sclerosis, but the same problems can arise with a syrinx or old trauma. Dorsal column stimulation is usually effective in controlling this pain.

Thalamus

Vascular lesions in the thalamus may cause a contralateral distressing burning pain, often associated with hypersensitivity. This usually fades spontaneously but may last years and is sometimes the reason for suicide.

When the patient is examined there may be an elevated pain threshold in the affected territory but above this threshold the patient complains that the pain provoked by the examiner's pin is abnormally unpleasant and occupies a larger area than normal.

Further reading

FiELDS, H.L. (1990) *Pain syndromes in Neurology*. Butterworths, London.

Paraesthesiae

Again the patient's fear, usually this time of multiple sclerosis, may contaminate the story. The words used to describe sensory disturbance include pins and needles, numbness, tingling, burning, swelling and coldness. Simple pins and needles may be due to hyperventilation, or to peripheral nerve, posterior column, or central lesions. Other sensory symptoms may be more revealing. Thus an illusion of heat or of running cold water on the skin or a burning or searing pain implies a disturbance more likely to be in the spinothalamic tract than the posterior columns, whose damage is more likely to provoke complaints of a tight band around the limb, a feeling of swelling or bursting. Parietal lobe lesions may produce complaints of loss of a limb, unfamiliarity or heaviness, or the presence of sensory or motor deficit may be denied. The left side particularly may be ignored.

The paraesthesiae due to hyperventilation are episodic in appearance and are usually present in all the digits of both hands and around the lips. Overbreathing may be denied but the patient may complain of a sense of being unable to take a deep breath and an eyewitness may refer to much sighing. The neurological examination is normal in this context. It may be helpful to ask the patient to overbreathe in front of the examiner and so reproduce the symptoms. Explanation of the cause of the symptoms and some simple relaxation techniques may suffice to treat such patients. Faintness, dizziness, tightness of the chest and a faraway feeling, as well as paraesthesiae may be reported.

The pins and needles of a carpal tunnel syndrome (CTS) can usually be identified by their nocturnal occurrence (and their aggravation by using the hands and wrists) and their relief by hanging the hand over the side of the bed. Patients often describe a strategy of hand flicking in an attempt to relieve their pain. There may be some flattening and weakness of abductor pollicis brevis and some increase in two-point threshold over the tip of the index. Forced flexion of the wrist (Phalen's sign) and tapping the nerve at the wrist (Tinel's sign) may aggravate the pins and needles. Nerve conduction studies should be carried out to confirm the diagnosis prior to surgical decompression. Although the median nerve only supplies three and a half fingers, it is commonplace for these patients to insist that all fingers are affected until they are asked to observe closely when next symptomatic.

The paraesthesiae of an ulnar neuritis are also painful and occur in the little and ring fingers and the ulnar border of the hand. They may be provoked by flexion of the elbow and are commonly worse in the cold. There is usually associated pain in the ulnar border of the hand and over the medial aspect of the forearm. The patient may have discovered that the ulnar nerve at the elbow is tender. In general, though pain and paraesthesiae are helpful in localizing peripheral nerve lesions, the subjective area of disturbed sensation is often greater than the true distribution of the damaged nerve. Testing often also reveals a larger area of disturbance of appreciation of light touch than of pinprick.

Paraesthesiae in the hands and feet that are more persistent than those produced by hyperventilation may be due to a peripheral neuropathy. The toes and feet are often affected first, the fingertips perhaps being the only area affected in the upper limbs. The diagnosis is supported by depressed or lost tendon reflexes, e.g. loss of both ankle jerks and the finding of distal blunting to pinprick and diminished appreciation of light touch in glove and stocking distribution. If paraesthesiae extend above the knee, especially if the hands are normal, one should begin to suspect a central, i.e. spinal cord, lesion.

The pins and needles experienced by patients whose multiple sclerosis has produced plaques of demyelination in the dorsal root entry zone or dorsal column of the cervical cord are usually described as being painless, affecting all digits and associated with clumsiness due to the joint position sense loss. In this situation, flexion of the neck can cause electric-shock-like sensations in the trunk and limbs (Lhermitte's sign). Although this symptom is classically associated with multiple sclerosis, rarely it is associated with subacute combined degeneration of the cord, cervical cord tumours, and radiation myelopathy. Cervical spondylosis commonly causes sensory symptoms in the arms, usually clearly of root distribution (outer border of arm, thumb, index with C6, back of arm and middle finger with C7, inner border of arm and hand with C8, inner border of arm around elbow with T1). C5–6 lesions predominate, with osteophytes at this level encroaching on exit foramina causing C6 root paraesthesiae most often. Diagnostic reflex changes, e.g. loss of the biceps jerk and 'inversion' of the supinator jerk (p. 37), and local abnormalities of neck mobility with cervical pain usually allow discrimination from the CTS, although the two may coexist and nerve conduction studies may be necessary. The presence of X-ray changes is not conclusive, since 50% of normal subjects over the age of 50 have some osteophytic formation. Extension of the neck may aggravate symptoms or cause Lhermitte-like sensations, the so-called reversed

Lhermitte's sign, due to buckling of the ligamentum flavum into the already compressed cord.

Central lesions usually produce paraesthesiae of a hemi-distribution affecting one side of the face, arm or leg. If the lesion is in the cortex or capsule the trunk may be spared. Cortical lesions may only affect the angle of the mouth or part of the limb. If the lesion is in the thalamus, the trunk is more likely to be affected along with the limbs. If the lesion is in the brain stem, the side of the face affected may be opposite to that in the limbs due to the lesion being above the decussation of the sensory tracts from the limbs but below the trigeminal crossing. Focal epilepsy in the sensory cortex may cause a spreading sensory attack with pins and needles beginning in the hand, but then spreading up the arm and onto the face, for example. This can be difficult to discriminate from an ischaemic attack in the same territory. In the case of the motor areas, the positive symptoms of a discharging focus with twitching of the limb spreading to the neighbouring joints is more readily distinguished from the negative effects of ischaemia with pure paralysis. In the sensory modality the difference between positive numbness (epilepsy) and negative numbness (ischaemia) cannot be made.

Muscle weakness

Patients' terminology when referring to muscle weakness is highly variable. Some use words that superficially sound more likely to relate to sensory phenomena, such as heaviness, numbness, and deadness. Other difficulties imply weakness such as difficulty in lifting their feet over obstructions, turning keys or doorknobs, keeping soap out of their eyes, chewing tough meat, sucking through a straw, getting food trapped in the mouth, or a nasal speech. There are some recurring patterns.

Generalized weakness

Further enquiry may reveal that a patient complaining of weakness is really describing a feeling of mental exhaustion, and the problem is due to a depressive illness. If the patient insists that there is true muscular weakness, there are a number of possibilities to be considered. There may still be no true weakness (hysterical weakness) or there may be a disorder of upper motor neurones, lower motor neurones, the neuromuscular junction or of muscle itself (Table 2.4).

Table 2.4 Differential diagnosis of weakness

Lesion	Wasting	Fasciculation	Tone	Reflexes	Plantar	Sensation	Pattern of weakness
UMN	0	0	↑	↑	↑	↓ or N	UL shoulder abduction, elbow extension, wrist extension, finger extension and abduction LL hip flexion, knee flexion, ankle dorsiflexion and eversion
LMN	++	+	↓	↓ or lost	↓	Usual depending on cause	Root – local territory Nerve – local territory Peripheral neuropathy – symmetrical distal
NMJ	0	0	N	N	↓	N	Eyelids, eyes, jaw, face, palate, pharynx, neck, limbs: marked fatiguability
Muscle	+	0	N	N or ↓	↓	N	Symmetrical proximal

UMN = Upper motor neurone.
LMN = Lower motor neurone.
NMJ = Neuromuscular junction (myasthenia gravis).
N = Normal.
UL = Upper limb.
LL = Lower limb.

Due to hysteria

Hysterical weakness is strikingly variable, jerky, and often 'gives'. It is of course unaccompanied by changes in tone or reflexes. If the patient can, with encouragement, produce even a brief instant of full power in each muscle group, then no fixed deficit exists. The patient's performance may contain marked discrepancies. Thus he may be unable to lift either leg off the bed during formal testing but be able to walk. He may get up from a chair when officially unobserved but evince paralysis of the hip girdle muscles and the quadriceps. A foot drop 'on the bed' may disappear when walking. Well-groomed hair may contrast with an inability under examination to lift the hands above shoulder height. During flexion of the hip on the couch, the normal person extends the opposite leg into the couch to gain power. A hand discretely placed under the opposite heel or calf can sense this. If it does not occur (though hip extension is powerful when tested directly) one can conclude that the patient is 'not trying' to elevate the other leg. Contraction of antagonists is also frequently felt when testing patients with hysterical weakness.

There is a trap in this description of how to diagnose hysterical weakness. Patients with myasthenia gravis may have variable muscle strength and of course they show no change in tone or reflexes. Power may fail suddenly due to fatigue of neuromuscular transmission, and this often looks 'hysterical'. The development of ptosis during maintained gaze above the horizontal is usually conclusive, however. If in doubt electrophysiological tests, edrophonium (Tensilon) testing and measurement of the titre of anti-acetylcholine receptor antibody may be needed.

Due to muscle disease

The weakness of primary muscle disease is usually symmetrical and characteristically affects proximal limb girdle muscles. There is weakness around the shoulders and hips with much more normal strength of grip and without foot drop. The patients have difficulty rising from a low chair, combing their hair, putting a case on a luggage rack in the train, hanging out washing or reaching high shelves. They may have difficulty whistling, chewing and swallowing. Tendon reflexes are commonly normal but may be reduced. There are no sensory symptoms but muscle pain may be a feature.

There may be little weakness on the bed but the gait may show a side-to-side waddle like a duck due to hip girdle weakness (the hip drops on the side of the elevated leg due to weakness of the gluteus medius). The patient may be unable to rise from a deep squat or even get out of a chair. He may need to use his arms on the bannisters when climbing stairs. A very proximal distribution with no weakness detected on the couch is commonly seen in the myopathy of metabolic bone disease. More obvious difficulty using the shoulders and legs develops in the genetically determined muscular dystrophies and the myopathies of endocrine and other systemic disorders. Steroid myopathy often affects the legs more than the arms, and normally reflects many months of high-dose treatment. Weakness of the neck is seen in polymyositis, myasthenia, dystrophia myotonica (and motor neurone disease).

Muscle disease may be genetically determined (dystrophies), inflammatory (polymyositis) or metabolic. In addition, there are some congenital myopathies.

Muscular dystrophy

The genetically determined dystrophies are described in Table 2.5. They mostly show a slow onset and gradual progression of weakness. Best known of these is Duchenne dystrophy. It affects boys in early childhood who, having learnt to walk, show a clumsy waddle and have difficulty rising from the floor. They use their hands to press down on their knees to straighten up. Their calves look plump though weak (pseudohypertrophy) due to replacement of muscle by fat and connective tissue. The EMG records reveal small polyphasic potentials and serum creatine kinase (CK) levels are grossly elevated. CK levels can also help to identify the carrier female. The condition is progressive, with the unfortunate

Table 2.5 Muscular dystrophies

	Decade	Pattern
Facioscapulo-humeral	2–3	Face, shoulder, may have foot drop, mild
Limb girdle	1–4	Shoulder or pelvic first, deltoid often spared, same picture can be neurogenic
Duchenne	1 (sex linked: boys)	Pseudohypertrophy calves, elevated creatine kinase activity, severe weakness, some have reduced IQ
Ocular	2–3	Eyes and eyelids, eyes may become immobile but no diplopia, ± pharynx, neck, shoulder and face weakness
Dystrophia myotonica	2–4	Bald, cataract, testicular atrophy, distal weakness, myotonia

victims limited to a wheelchair in about 10 years and usually dead of respiratory complications by 15 years from the onset.

Facioscapulo-humeral dystrophy is often missed, since the mild weakness of facial muscles and the neck and shoulders is so insidious in onset that it may not be thought abnormal, even by the patient, for many years. Onset is usually in adolescence and the eventual disability modest and not life threatening. Eye closure is affected, and the face looks gaunt with a lack of mouth movement during an attempted smile. The lack of good fixation of the scapula means that on full abduction of both arms to the horizontal, the tip of the scapula rides up and is visible over the clavicle from the front.

Also often modest in severity, limb girdle dystrophy causes weakness confined to pelvic and shoulder girdles. Patients become weak as young adults, finding difficulty with lifting their arms above their heads, combing their hair, rising from a low chair, climbing stairs, etc. This syndrome may be mimicked by neurogenic conditions, and full investigation may be needed to distinguish the type of pathology responsible.

Rarer conditions affect distal muscles or affect ocular muscles. Ptosis and ophthalmoplegia without diplopia is associated with some facial or pharyngeal weakness in the genetically determined ocular myopathies.

Dystrophia myotonica

Dystrophia myotonica is found in some 5 per 100 000 of the population and is inherited as an autosomal dominant disease. Muscle weakness and wasting affects the face, neck and distal limb muscles. The gaunt face with snar-

ling smile and thin neck from loss of sternomastoids is made even more characteristic by frontal baldness and thick spectacles following cataract surgery. As well as baldness and cataracts patients often show a degree of mental retardation, hypogonadism, impaired glucose tolerance and cardiomyopathy. The other diagnostic neurological feature is of myotonia with difficulty releasing grip, especially in the cold. The patient has to unpeel his fingers, often with the help of the other hand. It is important to recognize the condition not only because its victims are at risk under general anaesthesia but also so that genetic advice can be given. Other causes of myotonia include myotonia congenita (in which there is hypertrophy of muscles in the young patient), acid maltase deficiency in a middle-aged person with attendant myopathic weakness of limbs and respiratory muscles, and hyperkalaemic periodic paralysis in which attacks of severe weakness occur.

Polymyositis

Inflammatory muscle disease may be idiopathic or may complicate neoplasm or connective tissue disease. A reddish skin eruption on the face, upper arms and trunk may accompany the muscle disease ('dermatomyositis'). The muscle weakness affects the neck and proximal girdle muscles which may be painful and tender. The rule of thumb that muscle disease produces symmetrical proximal weakness is occasionally broken. Myositis can be surprisingly focal. The ESR is raised in about a third of cases, the creatine kinase activity in about 90%. EMG findings are of small polyphasic 'myopathic' potentials plus fibrillations. Muscle biopsy (which must avoid sites of EMG needling) is diagnostic with necrotic fibres and foci of inflammatory cell infiltration. A search for an underlying carcinoma or lymphoma is appropriate, especially in males over the age of 50; and the features of connective tissue diseases like systemic sclerosis (scleroderma), systemic lupus erythematosis and polyarteritis nodosa should be sought. Anyone with myopathic weakness over the age of 30, who is not systemically ill, should be assumed to have polymyositis until proved otherwise. The differential diagnosis of myopathy and a raised CK level includes infective myositis, toxic myopathies, dystrophies, and metabolic myopathy.

Metabolic and other systemic disorders

Painless proximal limb girdle weakness may accompany a number of endocrine and metabolic conditions (Table 2.6). Muscle fatigue and weakness are common with adrenal insufficiency and hypothyroidism. The disturbance of muscle function in osteomalacia is likely to be missed unless the patient is examined in real-life situations such as climbing stairs and rising from a low stool. On the couch little or no weakness may be found, since it is particularly concentrated in very proximal muscles around the hip.

Treatment with steroids can produce proximal weakness, especially in the legs. Several months of high-dose steroids are normally needed to produce a steroid myopathy, though a few patients become weak after only a few days of intravenous therapy, for example for status asthmaticus. Chloroquine

Table 2.6 Systemic causes of muscle weakness

Thyrotoxicosis
Hypothyroidism
Cushing's disease or steroid therapy
Acromegaly
Sarcoidosis
Amyloidosis
Osteomalacia
Hyperparathyoidism
Alcohol
Remote malignancy
Drugs, e.g. chloroquine, clofibrate

and clofibrate are other potential causes of iatrogenic myopathy.

Alcoholics usually have a subclinical myopathy if biopsies are performed. Symptomatic muscle disease may develop acutely and be painful, or chronically when it is slower to respond to abstinence.

EMG studies in these toxic, metabolic conditions are less revealing than with polymyositis and dystrophies. Type II fibres are predominantly affected and they contribute less to the EMG recordings during voluntary sustained contraction.

Other muscle diseases

Finally, there are some rare congenital myopathies (sometimes classified as dystrophies) most with distinctive histological abnormalities by which they are known, e.g. central core disease, nemaline myopathy, myotubular myopathy. The patients have hypotonic muscles and are slow to learn to walk. Most of the conditions are very slowly progressive, although central core disease is non-progressive. Disorders of glycogen and lipid metabolism may also cause hereditary myopathies of early onset. Metabolic muscle disease may cause both pain and cramps after exercise (McArdle's disease, phosphofructokinase deficiency, carnitine palmityl transferase deficiency). Ischaemic exercise of the forearm muscles below a cuff causes excessive rise in serum lactate which is diagnostic. The differential diagnosis of muscle pain on exercise includes ischaemia — intermittent claudication — when there may be telltale abnormalities of peripheral pulses, although these may only be detected after exercise. Neurogenic 'claudication' describes exercise-produced pain in the legs due to lumbar root compression related to degenerative disc disease, often associated with spinal stenosis.

Due to myasthenia gravis

The distribution of weakness in myasthenia is characteristic, with ptosis, ophthalmoplegia, weakness of jaw and face, with nasal dysarthria, dysphagia, difficulty with neck muscles, respiration and limbs. An aide-memoire for the usually affected groups is to consider which muscles are active even when the person is at rest, since the hallmark of the disease is pathological short-term fatigue. The eyelids, extraocular muscles, masseters, muscles of facial expression, neck and respiratory muscles are all active virtually continuously so they might be 'expected' to show fatigue before others. Bilateral ptosis with weakness of the jaw will almost certainly prove to be due to myasthenia gravis.

Due to peripheral neuropathy

By contrast, the weakness due to a peripheral neuropathy is distal in distribution. Hands and feet show muscle wasting and weakness at a time when the shoulders and hips retain much more normal power. Wasted hands and bilateral footdrop may thus be seen when elevation of upper and lower limbs against gravity is normal. The tendon reflexes are depressed or lost, and sensory testing may reveal an equally distal 'glove and stocking' impairment. The acute post-infectious Guillain–Barré neuropathy is a little different, often showing quite striking proximal weakness, as may the neuropathy of porphyria. Patients with Guillain–Barré neuropathy or sarcoidosis may also have bilateral facial weakness, unlike other neuropathies (other cranial nerve involvement may be a clue to the cause of neuropathy with 3rd nerve damage in diabetes, 5th nerve in collagenoses, deafness in Refsum's, and the lower cranial nerves in diphtheria). Either the axons or the myelin sheaths of peripheral nerves may bear the brunt of the attack of different disease processes. The clinical sequelae are sometimes sufficiently distinct to be diagnostically useful.

Axonopathy

Here a metabolic lesion affects the whole axon, which dies back from the periphery. Symptoms usually develop slowly and sensory changes precede motor. The lower limbs are normally affected first, with early loss of ankle jerks and a glove and stocking distribution of sensory change. Nerve conduction stu-

dies reveal little or no slowing of motor conduction velocities with reduction in amplitude of sensory action potentials. The cerebrospinal fluid protein is normal. Recovery, if it occurs, is slow as it depends on regeneration of axons at 2–3 mm/day. Most neuropathies due to toxins or associated with vitamin deficiency are of this type (alcohol, vitamin B_1 or B_{12} deficiency, uraemia, porphyria, vincristine).

Myelinopathy

When the disease process affects Schwann cells with damage to myelin sheaths, the picture is a little different. Symptoms may develop rapidly because conduction fails as soon as one area of a nerve is demyelinated. Once again it is the lower limbs that are mostly affected but the weakness can be proximal and can involve cranial nerves. Motor changes predominate over sensory. All tendon reflexes tend to be lost and nerve conduction studies reveal marked slowing, often with a patchy distribution. The cerebrospinal fluid protein value may be raised if roots are affected. As nerve conduction recovers when just a few lamellae of myelin are restored, clinical recovery can be rapid. Hereditary neuropathies and particularly Guillain–Barré syndrome and chronic inflammatory demyelinating neuropathy are of this type as well as diphtheric neuropathy, that due to metachromatic leukodystrophy, paraproteinemia, and sometimes diabetes.

Mononeuritis multiplex

A third group of conditions produces a collection of individual nerve palsies: for example, an ulnar nerve palsy in one arm, a radial in the other and an asymmetrical foot drop due to lateral popliteal nerve lesions. If enough nerves are affected by focal lesions, a diffuse neuropathy is mimicked but the history may reveal the discrete onset. Infiltration or ischaemia of nerves usually underlies such cases of mononeuritis multiplex. Collagenoses, diabetes, leprosy, amyloidosis, sarcoidosis, leukaemias and lymphomas may cause this type of neuropathy, as (rarely) may serum injections.

Individual nerve lesions are usually due to entrapment (e.g. of the median nerve at the wrist) but occasionally they are ischaemic in origin when they develop acutely.

Differential diagnosis of the cause of neuropathy

The mode of onset may provide aetiological clues. Thus acutely evolving neuropathy may be seen with Guillain–Barré, infectious mono-nucleosis, porphyria, sarcoidosis, malignancy and/or following vaccination or exposure to toxins. Subacute development over weeks or even a month or two suggests myeloma or other malignancy. A chronic-sounding disease should suggest diabetes, renal failure, alcoholism, drugs, vitamin deficiency or paraproteinaemia but may also be seen with malignancy and sarcoid. Diabetes may cause an insidious chronic neuropathy but occasionally a subacute onset in a diabetic suggests vascular changes, for example in the development of foot drop or a proximal painful weakness of the thighs.

The predominance of motor or sensory changes may be helpful. Thus sensory features are most striking in the neuropathy of uraemia, alcoholism, leprosy, vitamin deficiency, endocrine abnormality, primary biliary cirrhosis, AIDS and sometimes myeloma and carcinoma. Motor findings predominate in Guillain–Barré neuropathy, hereditary neuropathies, infectious mononucleosis, lead poisoning, porphyria and hypoglycaemia. Though most patients have distal weakness, proximal weakness should suggest Guillain–Barré neuropathy or porphyria. Involvement of autonomic function should suggest amyloid, porphyria or diabetes. Ataxia due to neuropathy is particularly likely in the context of cancer, Sjögren's disease, Guillain–Barré, treatment with cis-platinum, and rarely with HIV or toxicity from pyridoxine. Other clues from associated features are shown in Table 2.7.

Due to upper motor neurone lesions

The weakness of upper motor neurone lesions has a selective diagnostic distribution as well as being associated with telltale increases in

Table 2.7 Associated features in cases of neuropathy

Neuropathy PLUS	Cause
Autonomic damage	Amyloid, porphyria, diabetes
Cerebellar deficit	Alcohol, vitamin E deficiency, carcinoma
Mental change	Alcohol, porphyria, carcinoma, B_{12} deficiency
Hepatosplenomegaly	Alcohol, amyloid, macroglobulinaemia, lymphoma, sarcoid, chronic liver disease
Lymphadenopathy	Carcinoma, lymphoma, leukaemia, sarcoid, macroglobulinaemia
Renal failure	Amyloid, myeloma, uraemia
Anaemia	Myeloma, uraemia, malabsorption, B_{12} deficiency, carcinoma, lymphoma, leukaemia, macroglobulinaemia, chronic liver disease
Pigmentation, skin changes	Leprosy
CNS involvement	Leukodystrophy, collagen diseases

tone and reflexes with extensor plantar responses. If both legs are affected, the term paraparesis or paraplegia applies. If all four limbs are affected by upper motor neurone weakness, the patient has a double hemiplegia or quadriplegia (Figure 2.11). If there is weakness of upper motor neurone type in the same arm and leg, hemiplegia, or hemiparesis is the correct designation. The latter two nouns tend to be used interchangeably though strictly hemiplegia should refer to total paralysis and hemiparesis to less severe weakness.

In the upper limb the weakness affects particularly shoulder abduction, elbow extension, wrist extension, finger extension and finger abduction. At each joint the antagonist movement is more powerful. In the leg the weakness affects hip flexion rather more than extension, knee flexion more than knee extension by the quadriceps and there is a foot drop with inturned foot due to greater weakness of dorsiflexion and eversion of the foot, than of plantar flexion and inversion. The patient may thus be able to stand on tiptoe but not on his heels.

Some books precis this information by saying that the weakness of upper motor neurone

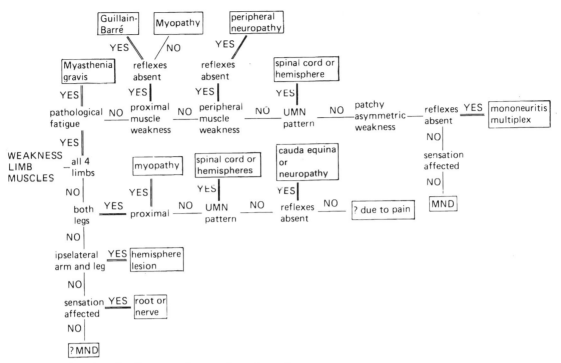

Figure 2.11 Flow chart for diagnosis of cause of muscle weakness.

lesions affects the extensors in the upper limb and the flexors in the legs, but this does not really help with the abductors and adductors at the shoulder, or eversion and inversion of the foot. It is easier to recall the chronic hemiplegic walking towards you with the curled up arm clamped to the side, and the circumducted leg scraping its inturned foot. Yet others refer to the pattern as being of the anti-gravity muscles, but it takes some mental agility to picture the patient as a quadruped, and then work backwards to define which muscles have an anti-gravity role.

Weakness in the arm

The upper motor neurone pattern has already been described. Weakness of the deltoid and a loss of dexterity in the fingers is the minimal sign and should be sought whenever the patient may have a hemisphere lesion, as part of the screening examination. Proximal

weakness in the limbs should raise suspicions of muscle disease such as polymyositis, lupus, sarcoid, paraneoplastic or alcoholic and other metabolic myopathies, or a dystrophy. In the upper limbs selective weakness of biceps and brachioradialis with sparing of deltoid and perhaps triceps suggests a dystrophy, as does a difference in the two heads of pectoralis. Muscle weakness (not of upper motor neurone pattern) with brisk tendon reflexes should suggest the myopathy of hypocalcaemia or hypercalcaemia and is seen in myasthenia gravis. Reflexes are often lost in affected muscles in dystrophies (though they may paradoxically be preserved in the calves affected by pseudohypertrophy).

Other causes of weakness around the shoulder are usually a reflection of a root lesion as in cervical spondylosis with damage to C5 or C6 roots (Table 2.8). There is weakness of the spinati, deltoid and biceps with C5 involvement, and with the additional involvement of the brachioradialis and supinator of the forearm in C6. With the former the biceps

Table 2.8 Cervical root lesions

Root pain	Weakness	Sensory loss	Reflex loss
C5			
Shoulder	Spinati, deltoid, rhomboids, biceps	Lateral upper arm	Biceps
C6			
Lateral forearm thumb and index	Brachioradialis, biceps, pronator/supinator, forearm, extensor carpi radialis longus	Lateral forearm thumb and index	Brachioradialis
C7			
Posterior arm medial aspect scapula	Triceps, wrist extension, extensor carpi ulnaris	Posterior forearm middle finger	Triceps
C8			
Medial side forearm	Finger flexion	Medial side forearm and little finger	Finger jerk cf. other side
T1			
Medial side arm	Intrinsic hand muscles	Inner aspect upper arm	–

jerk is lost; with the latter the brachioradialis reflex. Attempts to elicit the brachioradialis reflex may provoke finger flexion instead (so-called inverted supinator jerk). The features of individual peripheral nerve lesions are set out in Table 2.9 and the differential diagnosis of nerve and root lesions in Table 2.10. As an example of the exercise involved, one might cite the problem of distinguishing a high radial nerve palsy from a C7 lesion. Both cause weakness of the triceps and extension of the wrist. The radial nerve lesion also causes weakness of the brachioradialis and depresses its reflex (C6). By contrast, the C7 lesion spares the brachioradialis but may cause some weakness of flexion of the wrist.

In another context, victims of motor-cycle accidents may suffer traction injuries of the brachial plexus or avulsion of cervical roots. In both cases, the limb shows flaccid paralysis, perhaps of all arm muscles. If the lesion is in the distal plexus, however, two muscles

Table 2.9 Peripheral nerve lesions – upper limbs

Nerve	Weakness	Sensory loss	Reflex loss
Axillary	Deltoid	Lateral upper arm	–
Long nerve of Bell	Serratus anterior	–	–
Suprascapular	Spinati	–	–
Musculocutaneous	Biceps	Lateral forearm	Biceps
Radial (1) in spiral groove	Brachioradialis, wrist extension, finger extension, supinator forearm + triceps	Back of hand base of thumb	Brachioradialis
(2) upper arm		Base of thumb + Sometimes strip on back of forearm	+ triceps
Median at elbow	Wrist flexion, finger flexion, pronator forearm, thenar eminence	Lateral $3\frac{1}{2}$ fingers	Finger jerk (cf. other side)
Median at wrist	Thenar eminence only (abductor pollicis brevis)	Lateral $3\frac{1}{2}$ fingers	–
Ulnar at elbow	Flexor digitorum profundus (4,5) flexor carpi ulnaris, hypothenar eminence, interossei	Medial $1\frac{1}{2}$ fingers	–
Ulnar at wrist	Hypothenar eminence Interossei	Medial $1\frac{1}{2}$ fingers	–
Ulnar in palm	Interossei	–	–

Table 2.10 Root or nerve?

Problem	Differential diagnosis	Weakness	Sensory loss	Reflex loss
Paraesthesiae hand	C6 root	Brachioradialis	Lateral forearm	Brachioradialis
	Median nerve at wrist (carpal tunnel syndrome)	Abductor pollicis brevis	Distal to wrist crease	None
Wrist drop	C7 root	Triceps, sternal head pectoralis major, flexor carpi radialis	Middle finger	Triceps
	Radial nerve	Triceps, brachioradialis	Snuff box area	Brachioradialis
Weak interossei	C8-T1 roots	Interossei, APB, finger flexion	Inner border forearm, medial two fingers	Finger jerk compared with other side
	Ulnar nerve	Interossei, flexor carpi ulnaris	Distal to wrist crease, medial $1\frac{1}{2}$ fingers	None
Weak quadriceps	L3-4	Quadriceps, inversion foot	Anterior thigh and medial side shin	Knee
	Femoral nerve	Quadriceps only	Anterior thigh and medial side shin	Knee
Foot drop	L5	Hip abduction, hamstrings, foot drop, weak eversion foot, toe drop	Lateral side lower shin, dorsum foot	± ankle ± hamstring,
	Common peroneal nerve	Foot drop, weak eversion and toe drop	Lateral side lower shin, dorsum foot	None

whose nerve supply arises from roots proximal to plexus formation are spared, namely the serratus anterior and the rhomboids. If the lower roots are affected, a Horner's syndrome implies a proximal paravertebral injury to the T1 root rather than a more distal site of damage in the plexus per se. The distinction is of practical importance, since avulsion of the roots is irreversible whilst regeneration may reinnervate muscles when the damage is out in the plexus.

Weakness in the hand may be due to a cortical lesion, when global weakness of the hand is usually accompanied by some weakness of the deltoid and triceps and hyper-reflexia. In addition the loss of skill in the hand exceeds the simple loss of power in a way that is not seen with lower motor neurone weakness. Piano playing movements of the hand are slowed and clumsy, and the patient is unable to make discrete movements of individual digits. Brisk finger jerks may identify weakness in the hand as of upper motor neurone type. Lower motor neurone weakness of the

hand will often present with wasting of small hand muscles.

The wasted hand

The median nerve supplies the abductor pollicis brevis (APB) muscle at the lateral border of the thenar eminence which abducts the thumb at right angles to the palm. Isolated wasting of APB is seen with the carpal tunnel syndrome. Wasting of the interossei, obvious as prominent guttering of the back of the hand and of the web space between thumb and index and softening and flattening of the hypothenar eminence, with sparing of the APB is diagnostic of an ulnar nerve lesion. Global wasting of the hand is rarely due to a combined median and ulnar nerve lesion and usually due to damage to the T1 root, for example by a cervical rib or by cervical spondylosis. More extensive wasting in the arm occurs with syringomyelia and motor neurone disease and, when bilateral and symmetrical, with peripheral neuropathy.

Dropping things

The complaint that 'I am always dropping things' may reflect weakness when the objects are usually large and heavy. Dropping small objects on picking them up often proves to be due to a non-organic problem but dropping them after picking them up tends to be due to joint position sense loss in the fingers.

Weakness of the face

Unilateral weakness is either lower motor neurone (as in Bell's palsy) or part of a hemiparesis when upper motor neurone in type. The former shows equal weakness of upper and lower parts of the face, conspicuous difficulty with eye closure and burying of eyelashes. Emotional movements as when laughing are as defective as voluntary ones. The upper motor neurone version affects the area around the mouth more than the top of the face, and emotional movements may be preserved.

Bilateral UMN weakness can be part of a pseudobulbar palsy after bilateral strokes, for example, or with the UMN effects of motor neurone disease. Brisk jaw and facial jerks can be obtained. The latter are elicited by taking up cheek muscle between finger and thumb and tapping one's thumb with the tendon hammer. Motor neurone disease can also cause bilateral facial weakness of LMN type. Weakness around the eye should raise suspicions of myasthenia (with ptosis and diplopia) or ocular myopathy (no diplopia). If the whole face is also affected, dystrophia myotonica and facioscapulo-humeral dystrophy are possibilities.

Weakness of bulbar muscles

Bulbar weakness may usually be explained by motor neurone disease, myasthenia or poly-

myositis. Upper motor neurone signs or fasciculation suggest motor neurone disease, fatigue, myasthenia and an elevated CK polymyositis. Isolated weakness of chewing is usually due to myasthenia.

Weakness of respiratory muscles

Respiratory difficulty may result from brain stem-disease (stroke, motor neurone disease, or multiple sclerosis), high cervical cord lesions as after bilateral cordotomies for cancer pain or a high traumatic lesion, or from peripheral nervous system problems. The Guillain–Barré neuropathy can be complicated by respiratory muscle paralysis, as can myasthenia gravis. Polymyositis, dystrophia myotonica, and the myopathy of acid maltase deficiency are other possibilities to consider. Bilateral long tract signs would be expected with brain stem or cord disease, and arreflexia with Guillain–Barré. Dystrophies and other myopathies will be known about from the history. Myasthenia may present with respiratory weakness. Ptosis and a response to edrophonium will suggest the diagnosis. Polymyositis is the most difficult to pick up unless there is a rash.

Patients who fail to come off the respirator after an operation may have myasthenia, a mitochondrial myopathy, or after a stormy period with sepsis and multiorgan failure have developed a critical illness neuropathy.

Attacks of flaccid paralysis of trunk and limb muscles and sometimes of respiration but sparing eye movements suggests one of the familial periodic paralyses. That associated with high K+ levels is less severe, the attacks are shorter, the onset is early in life and there may be myotonia. That associated with low potassium levels is more severe and may be seen in thyrotoxic patients.

Weakness of the neck

If neck weakness predominates, myasthenia, polymyositis, systemic sclerosis, dystrophia myotonica and motor neurone disease are the most likely diagnoses.

Weakness in the leg

Upper motor neurone weakness initially causes some difficulty with hip flexion and dorsiflexion of the foot accompanied by impaired movement of the toes, hyperreflexia and an extensor plantar response. Such weakness may be part of a hemiparesis due to a lesion in the contralateral hemisphere or may be a monoplegia related to a smaller often cortical lesion. If both legs are involved, the responsible lesion will usually be in the spinal cord. The rare alternative possibility of bilateral cortical disturbance, for example from a parasagittal meningioma, will usually be indicated by focal epilepsy in the foot, papilloedema, drowsiness and dementia, as well as by brisk arm jerks.

The level of a cord lesion causing a paraparesis is judged by signs of local cord damage (reflex loss or muscle wasting) or by a sensory level. If the legs are affected but examination of the arms reveals no clues to a lesion in the cervical region, intercostal and abdominal muscles and the abdominal reflexes should be examined carefully. Perhaps paradoxical movement of intercostal spaces will reveal lower motor neurone signs indicative of a thoracic cord 'level' or the umbilicus will shift when the patient attempts to lift his head off the pillow. This sign (Beevor's sign) reveals loss of power in either lower or upper abdominal muscles and is again a sign of localizing value to the thoracic cord.

Spinal cord tumours may be extradural, intradural or intramedullary. Most extradural masses are metastatic carcinomas or lymphomas, and these produce back pain, root pain and a progressive paraparesis with late sphincter involvement. Haematomas and abscesses cause the same picture. Intradural tumours such as meningiomas and neurofibromas produce a slower tempo of progressive weakness and may produce strikingly asymmetrical changes. Intramedullary astro-

cytomas and ependymomas are less likely to cause local or root pain and more likely to produce sphincter disorders, local lower motor neurone signs and sacral sparing of sensory loss below their 'level'. Syrinxes cause a similar picture with suspended dissociated sensory loss and arreflexic muscle wasting locally (p.56 Figure 1.47).

Spinal metastases develop from primaries often situated in the lung, breast, prostate, or kidney, and lymphomas. In about half the cases the spinal lesion is the first manifestation of the tumour. Back pain with or without girdle pain and spinal tenderness usually precedes the subacute development of a paraparesis. Plain X-rays and CT scans usually show erosion of pedicles or collapse of a vertebra. The majority of cases affect the thoracic spine, though pelvic and colonic cancers are a little more likely to give rise to lumbosacral metastases, when root pain is usual.

Asymmetrical paraplegias are often due to multiple sclerosis, which has led to the suggestion that multiple sclerosis should be diagnosed if the patient complains of weakness in one leg but has upper motor neurone signs in two.

If all four limbs show an upper motor neurone pattern of weakness, then facial movements and the jaw jerk are examined with extra care. If normal findings result, then the likely cause lies high in the cervical cord between the foramen magnum and C3. If the jaw jerk is brisk or there is facial weakness, then brain-stem or hemisphere lesions are to be suspected.

A femoral nerve lesion causes weakness of the quadriceps with loss of the knee jerk. With a high femoral nerve lesion as caused by a haematoma in the psoas sheath, the iliopsoas may also be weak, so that flexion of the hip joint at 90° is also affected. L3–4 disc prolapse may also cause weakness of knee extension but also weakens inversion of the foot, enabling the distinction from a femoral neuropathy to be made at the bedside. The patterns of weakness associated with root and nerve lesions are set out in Tables 2.11 and 2.12.

Proximal weakness of the leg may be due to myopathy when symmetrical. This is very unlikely to explain a unilateral problem.

Table 2.11 Lumbar root lesions

Root	Site of pain	Weakness	Sensory loss	Reflex loss
L3	Anterior thigh	Hip flexion (iliopsoas) hip adduction, quadriceps	Anterior thigh	Knee jerk Adductor jerk
L4	Anterior thigh	Quadriceps tibialis anterior (inversion dorsiflexed foot	Anterior thigh	Knee jerk
L5	Lateral thigh	Hip abduction (glutei) hamstrings eversion foot (peronei) extensor hallucis longus	Lateral side shin dorsum foot	± hamstring
S1	Posterior thigh	Plantar flexion foot (mild) eversion foot (peronei)	Lateral side foot	Ankle jerk
S2	Posterior thigh	Intrinsic foot muscles	Back of calf	

Table 2.12 Peripheral nerve lesions – lower limbs

Nerve	Weakness	Sensory loss	Reflex loss
Femoral	Quadriceps	Anterior thigh medial shin	Knee jerk
Lateral cutaneous thigh (meralgia paraesthetica)	–	Anterolateral thigh	–
Obturator	Adduction hip	Inner aspect thigh	Adductor jerk
Common peroneal	Foot drop eversion foot	Lateral shin top of foot	–
Post-tibial	Flexion (plantar) foot	Sole of foot	Ankle jerk
Sciatic	Hip extension abduction hip knee flexion flail foot	Lateral shin sole of foot back of calf	Ankle jerk Hamstring jerk

Foot drop

A unilateral foot drop may be due to a lesion of the cortex (foot area), of the L5 root, or of the common peroneal nerve. The cortical lesion tends to produce a global weakness of the foot, and there will usually be slight hip flexion weakness (the upper motor neurone pattern) and an extensor plantar response to confirm its origin. 'Cortical' sensory loss may be found, e.g. difficulty with localization of a tactile stimulus. If there is an L5 root lesion, there will be weakness of dorsiflexion and eversion of the foot and extension of the big toe. More proximally, tone in the glutei may be reduced (which can be tested by palpation while the prone patient tightens his buttocks), hip abduction weak, and the hamstrings impaired. The hamstring and ankle jerk may be reduced. Sensory loss will be over the lateral border of the lower leg. Foot drop from a common peroneal nerve lesion combines weakness of dorsiflexion of foot and toes with weakness of eversion of the foot plus an area of sensory impairment or loss over the lateral border of the leg below the knee and dorsum of the foot. There is no proximal weakness, the reflexes are normal, and the plantar response is a normal flexor one.

Sciatic nerve damage, for example from a misplaced injection, causes weakness of all movements in the leg except hip flexion, knee extension and adduction of the thigh (femoral and obturator nerves). The ankle jerk is lost, and sensory loss affects the front of the leg laterally, the foot and the back of the calf.

Does the patient have motor neurone disease (Figure 2.12)?

This rightly feared diagnosis presents with either upper motor neurone or lower motor neurone signs, or a mixture of the two affecting limb muscles or those supplied by cranial nerves. There are no sensory signs but complaints of muscle cramps are common. Prominent fasciculations sometime give rise to odd symptoms like a feeling of champagne bubbles under the skin, which may be misconstrued as sensory in origin. Eye muscles and the sphincters are rarely if ever affected, and only terminally.

Fasciculation is common especially in the deltoid, pectoralis major and first dorsal interosseus muscle. Isolated fasciculation in the calves is usually physiological but may cause alarm, usually in medical graduates! It is only when fasciculation is widespread (e.g. tongue and both upper and lower limbs) and accompanied by weakness that motor neurone disease becomes highly likely. The combination of lower motor neurone signs in the upper limbs, e.g. wasted hands, and upper motor neurone signs in the legs should prompt the search for a cervical cord lesion before a diagnosis of motor neurone disease. A combination of lower motor neurone and upper motor neurone signs in the same limb, however, or in the same muscle (brisk reflexes in a wasted muscle) is suspicious of motor neurone disease. Eventually the lower motor neurone

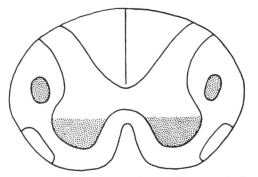

Figure 2.12 Motor neurone disease affects anterior horn cells with focal wasting, fasciculation and weakness, and the corticospinal tract with upper motor neurone signs but no sensory changes.

signs become generalized, when they must be distinguished by nerve conduction tests from a motor neuropathy. Tendon jerks are usually retained. The abdominal jerks tend to be retained later than in any other cause of paraparesis, in contrast with multiple sclerosis, for example, where they are lost very early. If only upper motor neurone signs are detected, the possibility of an intracranial lesion or spinal cord compression must always be considered.

When the presentation is with asymmetrical limb wasting and weakness progressing to a generalized lower motor neurone picture, the condition is called progressive muscular atrophy. When upper motor neurone signs are also evident, the mixed picture is called amyotrophic lateral sclerosis. If bulbar involvement is of lower motor neurone type, the name bulbar palsy is used; when of upper motor neurone type, pseudobulbar palsy.

The prognosis is better for younger subjects with limb involvement, though only about a third survive 5 years. There is as yet no known treatment.

Hemiplegia

Weakness of one arm and the leg on the same side, when of upper motor neurone pattern, is called hemiplegia or hemiparesis. A hemiplegia may result from damage to corticospinal and associated motor pathways from the motor strip to the cervical enlargement. The clinical examination provides localizing clues. If a hemiparesis is due to a high cervical cord lesion, e.g. at the foramen magnum or C1–3, then bilateral signs can be expected. The cord is small, and it is unlikely that a lesion there will produce motor tract damage confined to one side. The contralateral plantar response is likely to be extensor, therefore. The jaw jerk will be normal, demonstrating that the bilateral upper motor neurone signs do not originate higher than the cord, though this rule is not completely reliable. There will be no cranial nerve lesions, no visual field defect, no history of epilepsy, and no neuropsychological problem (Table 2.13). Shoulder shrugging and head turning will be normal.

Table 2.13 Regional localization

Hemisphere	Headache, personality change, epilepsy, cognitive defect, dysphasia, visual field defect
Brain stem	Diplopia, vertigo, nystagmus, ophthalmoplegia, ataxia, long tract signs, crossed sensory loss or facial weakness
Spinal cord	Spinal and/or root pain, sphincter disturbance, bilateral long tract signs, sensory/motor level

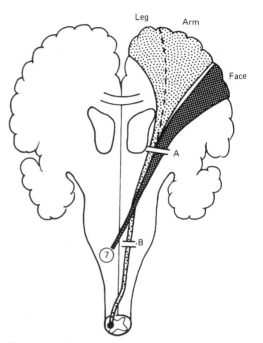

Figure 2.13 Lesions in the brain stem causing hemiplegia. A = Face, arm or leg hemiplegia. B = Face spared or weak on opposite side (lower motor neurone).

If the causative lesion is in the brain stem, then there may be cranial nerve signs such as weakness of turning of the head to the non-affected side, wasting of one side of the tongue, crossed sensory loss with numbness of the face contralateral to the affected limbs, dysarthria, diplopia, nystagmus or dysconjugate eye movement. Gaze paresis to the unaffected side may cause a deviation of the eyes at rest towards the affected limbs that cannot be overcome by the doll's head manoeuvre or caloric stimulation. Facial weakness may be on the opposite side to the hemiplegia and of lower motor neurone type (Figure 2.13). There will be no neuropsychological deficit and no field defect, but there may be limb ataxia or gait ataxia from involvement of cerebellar connections.

When the hemiparesis is due to a hemisphere lesion, the only cranial nerve abnormalities that may be encountered are of weakness of conjugate eye movement towards the affected limbs, and facial weakness on the same side as the weakened limbs. Confirmation comes from finding a visual field defect (homonymous hemianopia or quadrantanopia or inattention in a half field) and neuropsychological deficit, e.g. dysphasia with a left-sided lesion causing right hemiparesis, or neglect and denial with visuospatial difficulties in a right-sided lesion.

Small deep capsular lesions may cause hemiparesis with no psychological deficit, visual field or sensory change — the so-called pure motor hemiparesis. Slightly larger, more posterior lesions may cause hemisensory disturbance as well as hemiparesis. Larger lesions still will cause additional visual field defects and dysphasia if on the left. Massive dominant hemisphere damage causes deviation of the eyes 'looking at the damaged hemisphere', hemiplegia, hemisensory loss, hemianopia and global dysphasia.

A monoparesis, e.g. of an arm of upper motor neurone type, is usually cortical in origin. A monoparesis of a leg may rarely arise from a cord lesion but is also seen with cortical damage.

Cause of hemiparesis

The commonest cause of a hemiparesis is a cerebral infarct. The symptoms and signs may be sufficient to define the vascular territory of the ischaemic event. If the ischaemic area is in the central 'core' territory of the anterior cerebral artery, the clinical picture is of weakness of the contralateral leg and shoulder with the arm and hand relatively spared. Ischaemia in the distribution of the anterior cortical branches of the middle cerebral artery produces sensory and motor deficit in the contralateral face, arm and leg with Broca aphasia if the dominant hemisphere is involved. The leg is often least affected. If the territory affected is that of the posterior branches of the middle cerebral artery, sensory changes predominate with only minimal weakness. There is, however, a hemianopia and, if the dominant side is involved, a Wernicke aphasia. If the small penetrating branches of the middle cerebral artery are responsible for ischaemia of the internal capsule, there is weakness and/or sensory disturbance on the contralateral face, arm and leg to equal degree. Ischaemia in the posterior cerebral artery distribution often produces an isolated hemianopia. Carotid artery occlusion often causes the same deficit as middle cerebral artery occlusion, since collateral supply often salvages the territory of the anterior cerebral artery.

Occlusion of small penetrating vessels by emboli or more usually in response to the damaging effects of small vessel disease due, for example, to sustained hypertension may cause small deep infarcts in the basal ganglia, capsule or pons. Such lacunar infarcts cause restricted deficits; for example, a pure motor hemiplegia without sensory loss or pure hemisensory lesion without weakness, a combination of dysarthria and a clumsy hand, or ipsilateral ataxia and weakness, especially in the foot.

Further reading

PATTEN, J. (1996) *Neurological Differential Diagnosis*. 2nd edn. Elsevier, London.

ROWLAND, L.P. (1991) Amyotrophic lateral sclerosis. *Adv. Neurol.*, 56. Raven Press, New York.

Has the patient got Parkinson's disease?

Most patients with parkinsonism present with the development of tremor, commonly at first limited to one hand. The differential diagnosis of tremor is considered elsewhere, but the features suggesting that it is due to Parkinson's disease include worsening at rest, a pill-rolling movement of thumb against fingers, its appearance when walking and other early features of the disease. Thus a hint of increased tone, a lack of arm swing or loss of spontaneous facial gestures are all suspicious. Sometimes the tremor occurs in isolation for up to 2 years before it is clear that the patient has Parkinson's disease.

Many conditions may be suspected at the beginning. A patient's complaints of difficulty in using his hands or of walking slowly may be misconstrued as the effects of cervical spondylosis or a carpal tunnel syndrome. Unilateral slowing and rigidity and difficulty in skilful use of the hand may mimic the hemiparesis of a hemisphere tumour or stroke. Pain in the limbs may be misconstrued as indicative of a radiculopathy or carpal tunnel syndrome. A frozen shoulder may prove to be the first sign of emerging hemi-parkinsonism. Some patients describe a dystonic posturing of the foot with clawing of the toes which points to a basal ganglion problem rather than a cortical one, and this helps in the last distinction. Postural disturbance can also be useful in early diagnosis. The flexed posture of advanced parkinsonism may not be present but there may be a scoliosis associated with hemi-parkinsonism. The patient may describe a telltale hesitancy when walking through doorways or a reduction in size of their handwriting. Occasionally a writer's cramp turns into Parkinson's disease. (More usually this is a self-contained dystonic manifestation which is frustratingly difficult to treat. Most drug regimens fail, and patients end up writing with the other hand or learning to type.) The impassive face of early parkinsonism may be misconstrued as the effects of depression, with infrequent blinking and little play of emotion in the expression.

As Parkinson's disease progresses, the tremor spreads to affect the tongue, lips or chin, the foot as well as the hand, and it becomes bilateral. Rigidity becomes easy to elicit and the combined tremor and rigidity gives the feel of a ratchet or cogwheel when the wrist is flexed and extended. Rigidity may be felt in the neck and trunk. Slowing of finger movements becomes marked, the patient's voice becomes quiet and mumbling, his posture and gait stooped and shuffling. He walks with little or no arm swing, with small steps as though his feet were glued to the floor. He freezes and makes little stuttery movements before he can start to walk. He falls from slowness of movement and from loss of righting reflexes that make him vulnerable in a jostling crowd. Bladder instability may develop, and a modest degree of mental deterioration supervenes in up to a third. Despite modern treatment, patients still die of Parkinson's disease, usually of pneumonia or a pulmonary embolus. Post-encephalitic Parkinson's disease is characterized by a stable rather than progressive condition, and by seborrhoea and ocular crises in which the eyes become stuck in full upgaze for minutes on end.

The majority of sufferers from Parkinson's disease have loss of dopaminergic neurones in the substantia nigra of unknown cause. In the Steele–Richardson–Olszewski syndrome, a parkinsonian-like rigidity affects the neck and trunk and, to a lesser extent the limbs. The head is extended rather than flexed, the brow lined rather than impassive and there is early dementia. The limb changes are symmetrical. The crucial distinguishing feature, however, is the patient's inability to look up or down, though movement of the head can still produce vertical gaze through vestibular reflex pathways. This 'supranuclear' difficulty with down gaze leads to falls on stairs and 'messy' eating. Parkinsonian slowness and rigidity may also be encountered in some atrophic conditions affecting the brain stem and be associated, for example, with cerebellar deficit and pyramidal signs (olivo–pontocerebellar atrophy) or autonomic damage (Shy–Drager syndrome in which the urethral sphincter is denervated and the patients have incontinence, postural hypotension and impaired sweating). In striatonigral degeneration, parkinsonism is accompanied by pyramidal signs and laryngeal stridor.

Phenothiazines may cause rigidity and slowness, as well as tremor, so the drug history of all patients showing parkinsonian features must be assessed carefully. The changes are reversible. In the majority of subjects given phenothiazines, parkinsonism develops after a few weeks or months. (Acute reactions to phenothiazines and metoclopramide include dramatic dystonic posturing which may mimic tetanus, with neck retraction and limb rigidity

or even decerebrate posturing. Parenteral anticholinergic preparations rapidly reverse the condition. Late complications of phenothiazines and some butyrophenones include writhing movements of tongue, mouth, face and neck (so-called tardive dyskinesia). This tends to continue despite stopping medication.

Gait disorder

Walking may be impaired by breathlessness, general fatigue (e.g. anaemia), arthritis, pain, etc. but the patient is usually well aware of these problems.

Primary gait disorders of neurological origin may be recognizable from the associated findings on the couch, or by the character of the abnormal gait (Table 2.14). Patients with upper motor neurone lesions affecting one leg (e.g. hemiplegia) drag the affected leg, abducting it in an arc with an inverted toe scraping the ground. The toe of the one shoe wears out. The difficulty is clearly due to a problem of lifting due to weak hip flexion, knee flexion and dorsiflexion and eversion of the foot. The appearance and sound of the gait are characteristic. Associated spasticity, brisk reflexes and an extensor plantar response confirm the conclusion based on watching the gait. Bilateral upper motor neurone involvement of the legs from a cord lesion produces a stiff-legged small stride pattern, often with associated ataxia when due to multiple sclerosis, and often with a tendency for the legs to cross (scissoring). Scissoring seems particularly common with hereditary spastic paraplegias.

The ataxic gait due to cerebellar lesions shows irregular foot placement, a wide base and obviously impaired balance. There may or may not be associated difficulty with sitting balance and limb co-ordination.

The peripheral muscle weakness of a peripheral neuropathy causes bilateral foot drop. The weak feet are slapped onto the floor; and

Table 2.14 Gait disorder

UMN unilateral	Hemiplegia	One leg dragged, circumducted with the toe scraping the ground and a stiff knee. O/E unilateral spasticity, weakness, hyperreflexia, plantar ↑
UMN bilateral	Spastic diplegia or paraplegia	Stiff jerky gait with tilted pelvis, may scissor, both feet scraped on ground, delayed flexion. O/E bilateral spasticity increased reflexes, plantars ↑ ↑
LMN unilateral	Root or peripheral nerve lesion	Foot drop, knee lifted high as toe trails on floor. O/E foot drop ± loss ankle jerk and sensory change
LMN bilateral	Peripheral neuropathy	Bilateral high steppage. O/E peripheral weakness and reflex loss
Muscle disease	Myopathy	Waddling gait, difficulty rising from squat. O/E proximal weakness
Sensory loss	Posterior column	Unsteady, irregular placement feet, high steppage, slapping or stamping of feet, balance worse in dark with eyes closed. O/E impaired joint position sense, Romberg positive
Cerebellar loss	Ataxia	Staggering wide base even with eyes open, lurch from side to side, veers off course. O/E ataxia limbs ± dysarthria nystagmus
Extrapyramidal	Parkinson's	Small steps, shuffling, flexed posture, lack of arm swing, festination. O/E rigidity, bradykinesia and tremor
Lacunar state	Small-vessel disease	'Marche à petit pas' but unlike parkinsonian, upright posture and normal or exaggerated arm swing. O/E mild bilateral UMN signs, may be demented
Apraxic	Communicating hydrocephalus	Hesitant, irregular steps, looks as though forgotten how to walk. O/E can make pedalling movements on couch, may be dementing, incontinent
Hysteria		Exaggerated slowness or staggering without injury – risking falls, elaborate balancing movements with arms and trunk. O/E no signs

O/E = on examination.

the gait, like the unilateral scraping of a hemiplegic walk, can often be diagnosed on hearing the patient coming down the corridor. The knees are lifted high to clear the toes from the ground.

A high steppage combined with ataxia indicates posterior column loss and is seen with tabes dorsalis and sometimes with early cord compression.

The gait disorder of Parkinson's disease is associated with a flexed position of the head and body and loss of arm swing. The patient takes little steps and may have great difficulty starting (freezing) or negotiating obstacles like doorways. They may be unable to prevent their pace increasing (festination). They may, however, be able to make a full stride to step over an obstacle.

A rather similar reduction in stride length also happens with diffuse cerebrovascular disease (marche a petit pas). Here there is less flexion and the arms are usually swinging in rather an exaggerated way. Elderly subjects often show a shuffling, rather unsteady gait that is often due to both vascular disease of the brain and cervical spondylotic myelopathy, compounded by osteoarthritis of the hips and mild peripheral neuropathy or impaired labyrinthine function!

Fatigue

Most patients complaining bitterly of listlessness, loss of energy and fatigue will have an affective disorder, and these somatic complaints will respond to treatment of their underlying depression. The patient may deny depression, especially if they are challenged as soon as the examiner hears the presenting complaint. Although this may be the most realistic hypothesis to generate at the outset, it is better to allow the interview and the rapport to develop before broaching what is a sensitive issue. It is useful to pursue this possibility more obliquely with enquiries over diurnal changes in symptoms, the effect of rest on the problem, changes in appetite and sleep pattern, etc. and then to ask whether the problem has led to the patient feeling in low spirits.

These same complaints can, of course, be due to systemic illnesses such as anaemia, leukaemia, lymphoma, carcinoma, renal failure, AIDS, or cardiac decompensation, so a full exploration of routine questions and a careful general examination are necessary together with appropriate blood tests, chest X-ray, etc.

Excessive fatigue may be due to neurological dysfunction. It is prominent in a few conditions. Firstly, the weakness of the legs due to spastic paraparesis in multiple sclerosis is often strikingly related to exercise. The patient may have little weakness 'on the bed' and few symptoms at rest but be disabled by reduced exercise tolerance. As they walk their legs feel heavier and drag and they feel generally exhausted. Similar deterioration may occur in hot weather, or after a hot bath due to the failure of demyelinated tracts to conduct fast trains of impulses at higher temperatures.

A similar complaint of weakness of the legs coming on while walking is characteristic of lumbar canal stenosis. The patients, usually middle-aged males, have a narrowed lumbar canal due to spondylosis. As they walk the normal lumbar lordosis increases, increasing pressure on lumbar roots resulting in weakness, e.g. a foot drop or paraesthesiae and numbness. Symptoms may be reproduced by standing with exaggerated extension of the lumbar spine. Cycling can be easier for the patient because of the flexed lower spine. The most useful procedure is to examine the patient after he has walked to the point of symptoms. A foot drop may have developed or an ankle jerk may have disappeared. MRI or CT scanning of the lumbar canal is diagnostic and a laminectomy may be indicated.

Muscle weakness with striking fatiguability is of course the hallmark of myasthenia gravis.

The patient is usually aware of being at his strongest on waking or after a period of rest and of deteriorating rapidly with using particular muscles. Ptosis and diplopia progressively increase in severity through the day. The patient may be able to read the morning paper with ease but have to prop his eyelids up with his fingers to read the evening paper. Chewing on tough meat fatigues the jaw rapidly and the voice may become nasal after a long conversation on the telephone. He may become breathless, trying to talk to someone while walking side by side. The weakness of myasthenic patients may remit for months on end, mimicking the remitting and relapsing nature of multiple sclerosis, though the presence of ptosis and absence of sensory symptoms should alert one to the difference. When testing for pathological fatigue of muscles, it is worth testing the most symptomatic groups. Ask the patient to maintain gaze just above the horizontal for at least a minute. This will provoke increasing ptosis. If there is ptosis already see if it is momentarily lost during upgaze after downgaze which does not occur with other causes of ptosis. Get him to hold both arms outstretched. The weakness may develop suddenly or gradually, and recover after only a few seconds rest. Also test eye closure, the tongue, and neck flexion. The fatigue of myasthenic weakness is usually briefly overcome by an injection of edrophonium chloride (Tensilon). Single fibre EMG is helpful and high titre of antibodies to the acetylcholine receptor in the blood is diagnostic.

A degree of fatiguability with a partial response to edrophonium (Tensilon) is occasionally seen in polymyositis and motor neurone disease but the ocular involvement in myasthenia gravis and the long tract signs of motor neurone disease usually make the distinction easy. The Lambert–Eaton syndrome, usually a complication of small cell lung cancer, causes fatiguable weakness of the trunk and leg muscles with a dry mouth. Ptosis but not persistent diplopia also occurs. An absent limb reflex may reappear after a 10 second contraction of the appropriate muscle. The syndrome is due to antibodies to voltage gated calcium channels.

Some patients complain of muscle weakness and fatigue after influenza. Whilst these symptoms may be non-specific in nature, a post-viral myositis may be seen. Some metabolic myopathies such as McArdle's disease produce pain and weakness after exercise, sometimes with myoglobinuria. Exercise may also provoke weakness in attacks of familial periodic paralysis.

Further reading

LISAK, R.P. (1994) *Handbook of Myasthenia Gravis and Myasthenic Syndromes*. Decker, New York.

Bladder problems

Control of bladder function is critically dependent on an intact central nervous system. Normal bladder function can be viewed as consisting of two processes — storage and voiding. The neural pathways which affect both these patterns of behaviour lie in the brain stem: in the pontine micturition centres. Throughout life the bladder exists in its storage mode, switching to voiding at a socially convenient moment. Storage requires input descending from the pontine micturition centres through the spinal cord to sacral levels where the parasympathetic outflow to the detrusor muscle is inhibited. Other processes which are important in storage are an active relaxation of the bladder, giving it so-called 'compliance' and the maintenance of a relatively higher pressure at the bladder outflow by the active contraction of the striated muscles of the pelvic floor and urethral sphincter. It is probable that many 'higher centres' are important in maintaining the pontine micturition centre in its storage mode and although the full extent of these centres is uncertain, there are well delineated areas in the medial frontal lobes which are critical to continence. At an appropriate moment higher centres flip the bladder-controlling programmes in the pontine micturition centres from storage to voiding. The first recordable event in voiding is a relaxation of the striated muscle of the sphincter and pelvic floor, followed some seconds later by a rise in detrusor pressure. Thus voiding is achieved by a voluntary process of relaxation.

From the foregoing description it is logical to divide bladder problems by the site of the lesion into suprapontine, pontine, spinal cord, conus and cauda equina, and peripheral nerve lesions as shown in Table 2.15.

Abnormalities of bladder control in suprapontine lesions are characterized chiefly by a failure of storage. Voiding is normally co-ordinated. Patients can be demonstrated to have the condition known as 'detrusor hyperreflexia' in which the bladder develops uncontrolled rises in pressure at low filling volumes. This results in the symptoms of urinary urgency, frequency and possibly urge incontinence. There is, however, little specific or localizing in these symptoms and the laboratory findings, and this has led to considerable confusion in discussion over suprapontine lesions and incontinence. All too often in the frail elderly and patients with Alzheimer's disease, incontinence is attributed to cerebral causes with little positive proof that this is indeed the mechanism. A smooth muscle disorder of the detrusor could produce the same clinical picture. Except for well described areas of importance in the medial frontal lobes, surprisingly little is known about the cortical or suprapontine control of the bladder.

Patients with brain-stem and mid-brain lesions may have disorders of bladder function due to involvement of the pontine micturition centre or their connections. Patients with such lesions may have both disorders of storage and voiding but often these symptoms go unnoticed in the context of life-threatening neurological disorders. An internuclear opthalmoplegia may be an indication that there is pathology at sites in the brain stem close to those which control bladder function.

Spinal cord lesions are the commonest cause of neurogenic bladder problems. Interruptions of connections between the pons and the sacral cord cause both disorders of storage (i.e. detrusor hyperreflexia) as well as disorders of voiding. Characteristically, when

Table 2.15 Bladder problems

Site of Lesion	Dysfunction	Aetiology	Neurological Signs
Suprapontine	Preserved co-ordination between detrusor and sphincter but detrusor hyperreflexia	Hydrocephalus CVA Parkinson's Frontal tumour Dementia	– Apraxic gait – Pseudobulbar palsy – Tremor, rigidity, etc – Grasp reflexes – Primitive reflexes
Pontine	Detrusor hyperreflexia or retention	Multiple sclerosis Pontine infarct or tumour	) INO))
Spinal cord (suprasacral)	Dyssynergia between detrusor and sphincter. Retention during acute spinal shock then detrusor hyperreflexia	Trauma Multiple sclerosis vascular, myelitis, cervical spondylosis	) Spastic paraparesis) or quadriparesis))
Cauda equina	Detrusor areflexia and denervated sphincter. Lack of desire to void. Incomplete emptying.	Injury Central PID Tumour, herpes zoster, sacral agenesis	) Root signs) Perineal sensory) loss) Loss anal reflex
Peripheral nerve lesions	Reduced sensation to residual urine, later areflexia, retention, void by abdominal straining	Small fibre neuropathy Diabetes Radical hysterectomy Abdomino-perineal resection of rectum	) Autonomic failure) Absent ankle jerks

INO = Internuclear Ophthalmoplegia
PID = Prolapsed Intervertebral Disc

the detrusor muscle contracts at a low volume, the urethral sphincter contracts simultaneously. This disorder is known as 'detrusor sphincter dyssinergia'. There are several consequences of this disorder: one is that abnormally high intervesical pressures can develop, causing reflux up the ureters and thus renal damage. Although this is a potentially serious condition in patients with traumatic spinal cord disease, it seems to occur uncommonly in patients with other causes of spinal cord dysfunction such as multiple sclerosis. The reason for this is not known. Due both to detrusor sphincter dyssinergia as well as the lack of normal excitatory drive on the detruser muscle during voiding, incomplete bladder emptying is common in spinal cord disease.

Conus and cauda equina lesions can result in a variety of urogenital disorders and impaired control of bowel function. Although an atonic bladder might be anticipated with damage to roots, the bladder changes seen following a cauda equina lesion are often unpredictable. Saddle anaesthesia is a prominent part of the symptomatology of patients with such a disorder.

Faulty bladder emptying can occur as a consequence of generalized peripheral neuropathy, particularly if it is of a type that affects unmyelinated nerve fibres. However, involvement of the bladder is unlikely to occur until there is other evidence of quite severe autonomic involvement.

An important step in investigating a patient with a suspected neurogenic bladder disorder, is a careful neurological examination. As a general principle, if a patient has no abnormality on neurological examination, expensive imaging techniques and sophisticated neurophysiological investigations rarely discover an otherwise unsuspected neurological abnormality. Table 2.15 shows the associated neurological findings for a lesion at each level. This is important both in terms of positively recognizing a neurological cause and also erroneously attributing bladder dysfunction to a neurological cause when in fact there is a urological abnormality. Radiological, neurophysiological and urodynamic investigations are discussed on page 144.

Management

Disorders of storage characterized by urgency, frequency and urge incontinence, and due to detrusor hyperreflexia are most effectively treated by anticholinergics. This type of medication blocks the parasympathetic innervation of the detrusor muscle, making it less over reactive. Currently, the most popular medicine is oxybutanine. The commonest side-effect is a dry mouth, impairment of accommodation only occurring at high dosages.

If there is any reason to suspect that the patient is not emptying his bladder, a measurement of the post-micturition residual volume should be made before starting anticholinergic medication. Because patients are often unaware of incomplete emptying, there is a case to be made for making this measurement routinely in patients with neurogenic bladder dysfunction. Incomplete bladder emptying can cause the bladder to contract reflexly thus exacerbating urgency and frequency, and anticholinergic medication given to lessen hyperreflexia may have an additional effect of impairing bladder emptying. Thus if a patient with incomplete emptying is treated with anticholinergics, his symptoms are unlikely to improve and will possibly even worsen.

The best management for incomplete bladder emptying is intermittent self catheterization. The patient learns to insert a disposable catheter into his bladder two or more times a day, eliminating any residual urine. Many patients can learn to do this for themselves, but some disabled patients, such as those with multiple sclerosis who have a tetraplegia as well as incomplete bladder emptying, may require their carer to do it for them. Patients or their carers are best taught the technique by specially trained nurses and can usually learn to do it as an outpatient. Continuous advice and reassurance should be made available in the first few months of using this technique but after a while most patients become competent and they find the benefits far outweigh the inconveniences.

With progressive neurological disease a stage is often reached at which the patient can no longer manage with intermittent catheterization and a permanent indwelling catheter becomes necessary. In these circumstances a suprapubic catheter providing continuous bladder drainage is a good option.

Further reading

FOWLER, C.F., BETTS, C.D. and FOWLER, C.G. (1992) Bladder dysfunction in neurological disease. In *Disease of the Nervous System* (eds A.K. Asbury, G.M. McKhann and W.I. McDonald), WB Saunders, Philadelphia, pp. 512–528.

Impotence

Much less is known about the neural control of sexual function than about neurological bladder function. Erectile dysfunction is, however, a prominent symptom in men with spinal cord disease. Preservation of psychogenic erections may occur in men with spinal cord lesions above the thoracic level, and reflex erections can occur in men with lesions below this level. Difficulty with ejaculation is also likely to be a problem with spinal cord disease. Conus and cauda equina lesions producing perineal sensory loss as well as loss of genital function cause major sexual difficulties in both men and women. It is as yet unresolved whether small fibre neuropathy alone is responsible for the high prevalence of impotence in diabetics, or whether the problem is due to a combination of small vessel disease and neuropathy. Diabetic men with erectile difficulties commonly have preservation of ejaculation. A neurological condition in which impotence may be the first and earliest symptom is multiple system atrophy. Why this should be is not known, but this symptom may long precede any other features of autonomic failure.

The introduction of intracorporeal injections of vasoactive substances to produce erection has transformed the management of this problem. Patients with neurogenic or psychogenic causes of erectile failure respond well to low doses of these substances, in contrast to men with arteriogenic impotence who may not obtain satisfactory responses. Men are taught to self inject using either papaverine or alprostadil, and are warned of how they should seek medical attention should they develop a very prolonged erection with a view to being treated with an antidote.

The only oral medication currently available which is thought to improve sexual performance is yohimbine. This is an alpha-2 agonist which has been shown in control trials to have some advantage over placebo in the treatment of impotence.

Many patients (and doctors) are shy about discussing sexual failure, and any individual with spinal cord disease, autonomic problems such as postural hypotension, or diabetes should be asked tactfully about this.

Further reading

BETTS, C.D., FOWLER, C.G. and FOWLER, C.J. (1992) Sexual dysfunction in neurological disease. In *Disease of the Nervous System — Clinical Neurology*, 2nd edn (eds A.K. Asbury, G.M. McKhann and W.I. McDonald) WB Saunders, Philadelphia, pp. 501–511.

DYSPHAGIA

The act of swallowing depends on a co-ordinated sequence of motor acts involving a number of cranial nerves and proximal muscles so is vulnerable to breakdown in a number of conditions.

The first phase involves chewing and sensing the food mass in the mouth (cranial nerve 5), spillage being prevented by lip closure (cranial nerve 7). The tongue then propels the bolus to the back of the mouth into the pharynx where its presence is sensed by the 9th cranial nerve. This triggers the reflex phase. The larynx is protected by being pulled up and tilted forwards (by cranial nerves 12 and 9) and by the epiglottis covering it (cranial nerve 10). The 10th nerve also elevates the palate to close the nasopharynx and prevent nasal regurgitation, and opens the hypopharynx and initiates oesophageal peristalsis.

Lesions of the 7th nerve cause spillage and of the 5th and 12th nerve cause difficulty in forming and throwing back the bolus. Loss of the 9th nerve prevents triggering of the swallow and with 10th nerve damage leads to nasal regurgitation or aspiration of mouth contents through the larynx.

Dysphagia is thus a problem with upper or lower motor neurone damage to the relevant cranial nerves or with muscle weakness due to myasthenia and myopathy.

Unilateral UMN damage as in acute stroke produces only temporary dysphagia but bilateral damage (pseudobular palsy) can cause persistent swallowing problems. Bilateral LMN cranial nerve lesions from nasopharyngeal cancer, malignant meningitis, Guillain Barré neuritis are more likely to cause problems than unilateral (e.g. from a mass at the jugular foramen).

The first essential when dealing with a primary complaint of dysphagia is to exclude a mechanical obstruction for example from an oesophageal cancer. In such cases swallowing is usually painful, the patients can localize the level of obstruction and solids are more of a problem than liquids. Next the lower cranial nerves are examined in detail though it is important to realize that a normal gag reflex does not guarantee a normal neurological swallow. ENT and speech therapy advice will usually be needed in the investigation and management.

3

Investigations

Electromyography (EMG)

The principal value of needle recordings of the electrical activity of resting and contracting muscle is to find evidence of denervation due to damage of the lower motor neurone (anterior horn cell or axon), and to distinguish between such neurogenic weakness and that due to disease of muscle fibres (myopathy, polymyositis, muscular dystrophy). The experienced electromyographer makes use of the appearance of the recordings on an oscilloscope and the accompanying sound on a loudspeaker. Quantitative methods are also available through the software on modern EMG equipment.

There are no diagnostic features of upper motor neurone weakness where muscle recordings show a pattern of motor unit activity indistinguishable from that of a normal subject making less than a full effort. The firing rates of individual motor units remain slower than that seen at full effort in normal subjects.

Lower motor unit damage, whether it is due to polio or motor neurone disease causing loss of anterior horn cells, or root or peripheral nerve disease damaging axons, produces telltale fibrillation potentials in the resting muscle (Figure 3.1). These small potentials recorded by concentric needle electrodes are the result of spontaneous firing of individual muscle fibres (fibrillation), which occurs when dener-

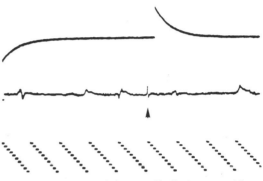

Figure 3.1 EMG record showing fibrillation potentials some nearer the needle tip (arrow) than others. Calibration in ms (lower trace) and 1 mV step (upper trace).

vation hypersensitivity affects the stability of the resting membrane potential of the muscle fibre. Further indications of neurogenic weakness emerge during contraction. Because anterior horn cells or axons are missing, surviving motor units are driven at higher rates than normal (Figure 3.2). If the tempo of the underlying disease is slow or chronic (e.g. poliomyelitis) surviving axons sprout and may reinnervate muscle fibres 'deserted' by their original connections. This leads to the development of larger than normal motor units with an increased number of muscle fibres connected to one of the surviving anterior horn cells. These are identifiable on the needle recordings by their increased size, complexity and duration (Figure 3.3). The distribution of denervation can of itself be diagnostic, for example when only muscles innervated by

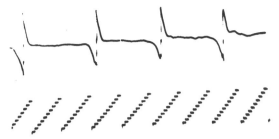

Figure 3.2 EMG record showing rapid firing of surviving motor unit in a denervated muscle. Calibration in ms (lower trace) reveals firing rate of 40–50/second – normally no more than 10–20.

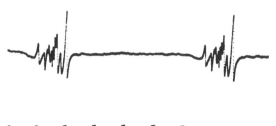

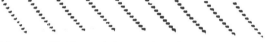

Figure 3.3 EMG record showing long duration polyphasic potentials in reinnervated muscle. Calibration in ms (lower trace). Peak to peak amplitude 2 mV (normal).

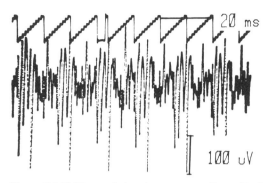

Figure 3.4 EMG record showing many small amplitude brief polyphasic potentials in myopathic muscle during modest effort. Note need to recruit many units because of reduced strength of individual units.

one nerve root are so affected and there are no abnormalities of nerve conduction, indicating a radiculopathy, or median but not ulnar muscles are denervated in a hand, suggesting an isolated median nerve lesion. Soft signs of denervation may be seen in muscles like the tibialis anterior, due to the frequency of trivial mechanical damage to its parent nerve at the knee, perhaps caused by sitting with crossed legs. In motor neurone disease muscle sampling may reveal telltale signs of denervation in all four limbs when perhaps weakness is only detectable in one.

By contrast, a myopathic muscle has a full complement of motor units but these are individually impoverished by a disease process that has damaged individual muscle fibres. The recorded motor unit potentials are small in amplitude, brief, and reveal their individual components by an increase in polyphasicity (Figure 3.4). At weak effort the oscilloscope

screen is full of potentials as numerous motor units are recruited, as they individually produce less force than normal. Patients with polymyositis may show a combination of myopathic potentials and fibrillation potentials.

Myotonia as seen in dystrophia myotonica and congenital myotonia is characterized by a waxing and waning frequency of muscle discharges which on the EMG loudspeaker sounds like a motor-cycle engine being revved up intermittently (Figure 3.5). Older textbooks use the analogy of a 'dive-bomber' — fortunately not a familiar sound.

Myasthenia gravis can be diagnosed from the behaviour of neighbouring individual muscle fibres connected to one and the same axon. If the oscilloscopic display is set to be triggered by the firing of one muscle fibre, the variable timing and success of neurotransmission to the second fibre can be documented. With myasthenic failure of some impulses to achieve the firing threshold of the muscle membrane, the second fibre sometimes does not fire ('blocking') and the interval between the firing of the two fibres varies ('jitter'). Such recordings need a special electrode designed for 'single fibre' recording (Figure 3.6).

EMG studies are thus indicated in the investigation of muscle weakness, suspected myopathies, myasthenia and patients with possible motor neurone disease. A confident diagnosis of motor neurone disease requires the demonstration of evidence of denervation of wide-

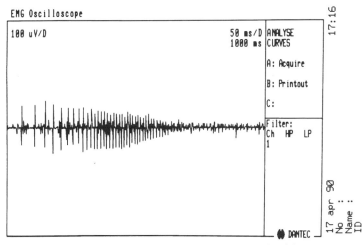

Figure 3.5 EMG record showing myotonia. The amplitude of the response waxes and wanes as does the frequency of the repetitive firing of individual fibres (50–150/s).

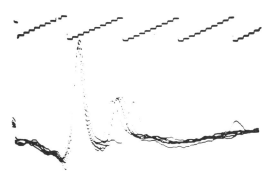

Figure 3.6 (a) EMG record from 'single fibre' needle electrode showing two muscle fibres firing. Calibration in tenths of a msec (upper trace). Note second fibre fires at a variable interval after the first which triggers the recording.

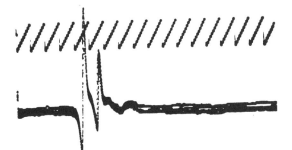

Figure 3.6 (b) Similar record from normal subject showing no jitter. The traces from the second fibre all superimpose in the same way as the first.

spread distribution demonstrably not due to peripheral neuropathy.

Nerve conduction studies

The measurement of the velocity of motor and sensory fibre conduction is normally supplemented by recordings of the amplitude of responses either in the nerve (sensory action potentials) or muscle (muscle action potentials) (Figure 3.7). Together, these parameters can reveal whether there is any evidence of disease of peripheral nerve fibres. The main technical trap for the unwary consists of not ensuring adequate warming of the limb, leading to falsely abnormal slowing.

Repetitive stimulation of a nerve causes a declining amplitude of muscle response in myasthenia gravis, and a temporary increase (200%) in the paraneoplastic Lambert–Eaton syndrome due to abnormalities at the neuromuscular junction.

Delayed conduction across an anatomical site of possible compression diagnoses an

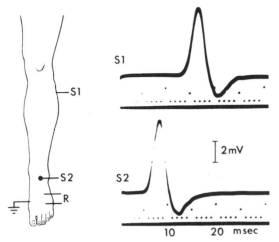

Figure 3.7 Set-up for recording amplitude of muscle response as recorded by surface electrodes over ext. dig brevis during stimulation of the common peroneal nerve proximally at the head of the fibula (S1 upper trace) and distally at the ankle (S2 lower trace). The difference in latency of response allows calculations of motor conduction velocity between S1 and S2 and changes in amplitude may reveal axonal loss (small response from both sites) or conduction block (smaller from S1 than S2).

entrapment neuropathy of, for example, the median nerve at the wrist (Figure 3.8), or the ulnar nerve in the cubital tunnel. As well as diagnosing the site of nerve damage due to trauma for example, neurophysiological tests

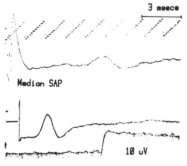

Figure 3.8 Sensory action potentials from a case of carpal tunnel syndrome. The upper trace shows a small delayed response over the median nerve at the wrist during stimulation of the index finger compared to a large earlier response over the ulnar nerve (lower half) during stimulation of the little finger.

can indicate the prognosis. Thus the amplitude of the muscle response may be smaller with stimulation of the affected nerve above a site of injury. If the amplitude is normal with nerve stimulation distal to the injury site, the local pathology in between must be of focal demyelination. The prognosis for early recovery after a single episode of damage, as when sleeping with the arm over the back of a chair leading to a 'Friday night ' paralysis of the radial nerve, is good in these circumstances. It only takes a few weeks for the myelin to be repaired. If the muscle action potential recorded from distal stimulation is small, or fibrillation potentials develop, then axonal loss must have occurred and recovery will require regeneration over the coming months.

Though a patient might have coincidental mechanical lesions of one carpal tunnel and one elbow, multiple focal conduction abnormalities are more likely to be indicative of a mononeuritis multiplex. This is especially likely to be true if the focal lesions are at sites other than sites of mechanical compression, e.g. the median nerve in the forearm, and the ulnar in the upper arm. The usual cause is a vasculitis, as in a collagen vascular disease. In some parts of the world leprosy is the commonest cause.

More generalized abnormalities are diagnostic of a peripheral neuropathy. If axonal damage predominates, as in most toxic neuropathies, then sensory action potentials are small and motor conduction velocity slightly reduced (from 50 to 40 metres per second, say) due to loss of some of the faster conducting nerve fibres. Abnormalities are more striking in the distal parts of the nerve. Muscle action potentials are small due to loss of motor units.

If demyelination is the main pathological process, as it is in some hereditary neuropathies for example, then conduction measurements show gross slowing: perhaps from 50 to 20 metres per second (more than a 40% reduction) and all sensory action potentials are unrecordable. Conduction abnormality may be striking in the proximal part of the nerve. Muscle action potentials may be dispersed due to differences in the time of arrival of a stimulus in different nerve fibres. The type of neuropathy as well as its presence can thus sometimes be inferred from the neurophysiological studies.

Special techniques are available to test conduction in the most proximal parts of peripheral nerves, e.g. at plexus level. 'F' waves (Figure 3.9) are recordings of muscle fibres contracting a second time after a distal electrical shock, due to retrograde stimulation of the motor fibre invading the axon hillock of the parent anterior horn cell and stimulating it to a discharge back down to the muscle. They are delayed in diseases like Guillain–Barré neuropathy which targets nerve roots and proximal parts of peripheral nerves, and with plexus lesions like those caused by a cervical rib.

Sensory action potentials (Figure 3.8) reflect the integrity of the sensory nerve fibres distal to the dorsal root ganglion (DRG). If the sensory root is damaged proximal to the DRG the distal fibre remains intact and the numb limb has normal sensory action potentials. If the distal fibre is damaged in the brachial or lumbar plexus, the sensory action potential is lost as the fibre degenerates. Conduction tests can thus be employed to help distinguish between root and plexus lesions, e.g. after trauma. Paradoxically, normal sensory potentials in a flail arm after a traction injury imply root avulsion and no chance of recovery, whilst loss of responses in the periphery indicates plexus injury with the potential for regeneration. (In the latter situation imaging is needed to see if there is additional damage at root level.)

Evoked potentials

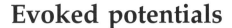

Sensory organs and their afferent pathways can be interrogated by scalp recordings of the small potentials that are time-locked to modality specific stimuli or are 'evoked' by such stimuli. Occipital EEG electrodes pick up small potentials (5 μV) in response to visual stimuli (visual evoked response – VER) (Figure 3.10), with abnormalities mainly of latency detectable with disease from the retina to the cortex. More complex waveforms result from click stimuli to the ears (brain stem auditory evoked response — BAER), and these are sensitive to disease of the cochlea or brain stem (Figure 3.11). Interpeak latencies are used to assess intrinsic brain-stem lesions. Electrical stimuli to peripheral nerves produce responses that are called somatosensory evoked potentials or SEPs (Figure 3.12). These detect changes in conduction from the peripheral nerve to the thalamus and cortex.

The main use of these responses in diagnostic neurology has been to detect clinically silent abnormalities in patients with a presenting illness affecting another part of the neuraxis. Abnormalities of visual evoked responses in a patient presenting with evidence of an isolated spinal cord syndrome, for example, have the same significance as finding clinical evidence of past optic neuritis: the multiplicity of lesions making multiple sclerosis the likely

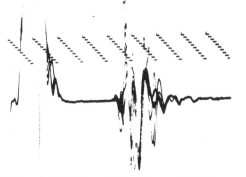

Figure 3.9 EMG record showing muscle 'M' response to nerve stimulation to left followed by 'F' wave responses some 43 ms later from antidromic stimulation of anterior horn cells by proximal conduction of the stimulus. Superimposed traces. Calibration in ms (upper traces).

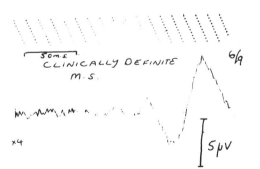

Figure 3.10 Visual evoked potentials from a patient with multiple sclerosis but normal visual function to bedside testing. The major deflection at 135 ms is much delayed (normal <120).

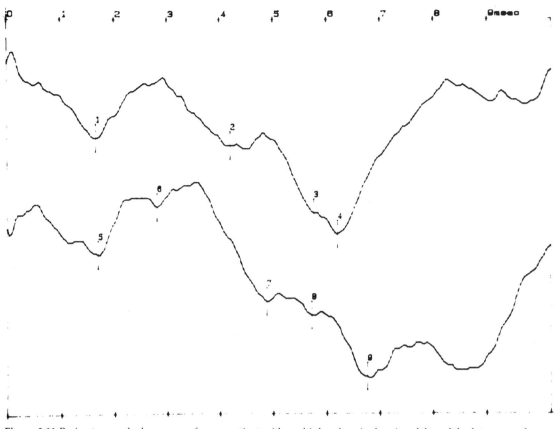

Figure 3.11 Brain-stem evoked responses from a patient with multiple sclerosis showing delay of the later wave forms in the left ear (lower trace) compared to the right (upper trace).

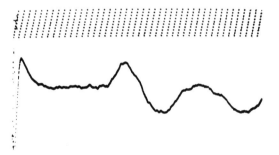

Figure 3.12 Somatosensory evoked potential. Small 5–10 μV response recorded by parietal EEG electrodes during stimulation of median nerve at the wrist. Latency approximately 20 ms. Calibration in tenths of ms (upper trace).

diagnosis. MRI evidence of multiple white matter plaques and the presence of oligoclonal bands on electrophoresis of the cerebrospinal fluid have to some degree usurped this role in the diagnosis of multiple sclerosis, but there are still circumstances when they remain useful. The patient who is intolerant of the rather noisy and claustrophobic environment of the magnet, or who declines a lumbar puncture can be investigated with a full battery of evoked potentials.

VERs are also useful in the assessment of other diseases of the optic nerve such as compression where amplitude is lost as well as latency prolonged, and of the chiasm where a comparison of the responses to stimulation of half fields can document subtle changes, even when fields appear to be intact.

BAERs are useful in the differential diagnosis of vertigo, helping to distinguish central from peripheral causes, and being particularly sensitive to the presence of an acoustic neuroma. BAERs can also be used to assess the cause and prognosis of coma. The responses are, for example, little affected by metabolic or drug-induced lowering of consciousness, whilst brain-stem structural disease causing coma will be associated with marked response abnormality. The preservation of BAER in the presence of a flat EEG implies a reversible metabolic (drug overdose) coma. In infants and unco-operative or retarded adults they can be used to assess hearing. In the operating theatre they may be used to monitor microvascular procedures in the posterior fossa, improving the safety of the operation.

SEPs, which are normally about $10\,\mu V$ in amplitude, serve a useful function in the search for evidence of central sensory pathway lesions in patients with sensory symptoms or signs. They are normal in cases of hysterical hemianaesthesia. They can aid in the assessment of plexus lesions and in the cervical rib syndrome for example, where delayed SEPs and 'F' waves may be the only clues to the cause of weakness and denervation in small hand muscles like the abductor pollicis brevis. Spinal SEPs are valuable guides to the safety of surgery, with continuous monitoring during surgery to detect potentially hazardous damage to the cord during straightening of the vertebral column.

Electro-encephalography (EEG)

Scalp recordings of the EEG remain valuable to clinical diagnosis and management despite the increasing sophistication of neuroimaging and the advent of evoked potential technology. The EEG provides an albeit brief view of the functional state of the brain which supplements rather than competes with images of structural changes. This is most clearly seen in the context of epilepsy.

Over 50% of patients with epilepsy have abnormal EEG records, and in about a third the changes are sufficiently specific to be of diagnostic help. In the case of petit-mal, a characteristic pattern of alternating spike discharges and slow waves at about 3 Hz occurs during the 10-second attack (Figure 3.13). Even if no clinical attack occurs during the recording, there is a very high chance that a second or two of 3-Hz spike and wave pattern

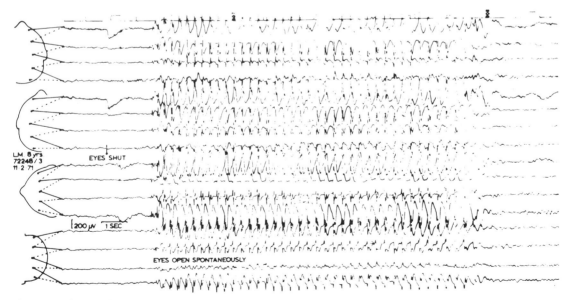

Figure 3.13 Sixteen-channel scalp EEG recording showing 3 Hz spike and wave activity during a petit mal attack in an 8 year old.

will be 'caught'. It may be triggered by having the patient hyperventilate.

Patients with grand-mal epilepsy are far less likely to show telltale spike discharges, though hyperventilation and photic stimulation may provoke them. In this context the real use of the recording is to detect otherwise unsuspected evidence of a focal origin for attacks (Figure 3.14). This is also true in the case of patients with temporal lobe epilepsy, when the symptoms of the partial complex seizure may not reveal which side is the source of discharges. A few spikes or sharp waves or even less specific slow waves from one temporal area (Figure 3.15) may be an important step towards the consideration of a possible surgical treatment for someone with drug resistant attacks. It also highlights the need

for neuroimaging (including MRI) if CT has been normal, and indicates where most attention should be paid when the images are reviewed. The actual imaging protocol can be tailored to the area thrown up by the discovery of lateralizing or localizing EEG changes. The most cost effective use of EEGs in epilepsy is to make frequent and detailed studies of a few patients with attacks that are difficult to diagnose and manage. The chances of picking up a tendency to paroxysmal discharges is increased after a sleepless night if the patient is allowed to go into the early stages of sleep. The combination of a waking and a sleep EEG reveals epileptiform activity in about 80% of adults with epilepsy. In practice, single records of every patient with any attack of dizziness, reduced awareness, etc.

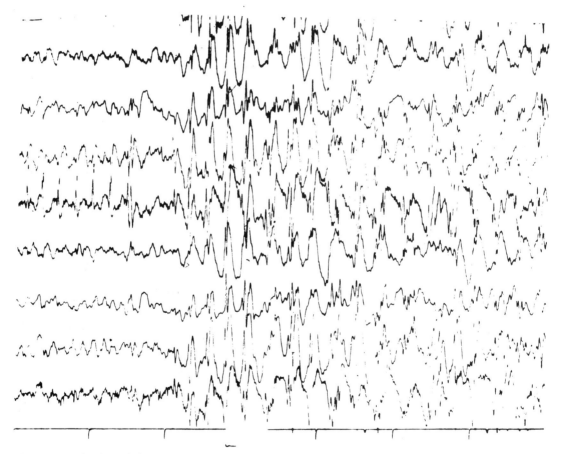

Figure 3.14 Eight channels from a scalp EEG record showing focal spikes (3rd and 4th channel from top) immediately preceding a generalized seizure. Calibration in seconds (bottom trace).

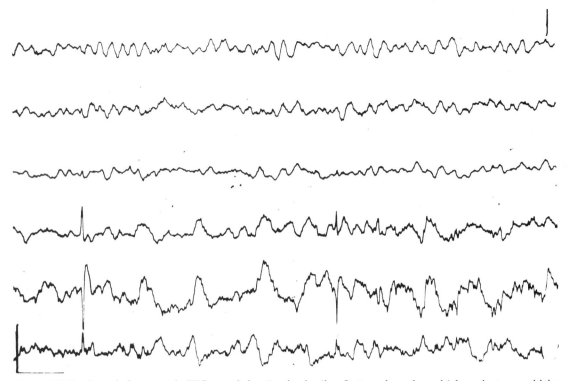

Figure 3.15 Six channels from a scalp EEG record showing focal spikes (bottom three channels) from the temporal lobe in the absence of clinical changes.

are usually requested, with too much reliance being placed on the negative predictive value of a normal 20-minute recording. It is important to remember that epilepsy is a clinical diagnosis and does not need EEG 'proof'. On the other side of the coin, an 'epileptic' record is occasionally obtained in an individual with no suspicion of any sort of epilepsy, when being screened for example in the armed forces. This only occurs in about 0.3%. In the case of petit mal with absence seizures, the situation is a little different. It would be unusual not to record some 3 Hz spike and wave activity in the child's record, and failure to precipitate it during hyperventilation virtually excludes the diagnosis. A staring attack with no accompanying spike and wave abnormality is not an absence seizure of petit mal type.

In particularly difficult cases, long-term EEG monitoring may be useful, especially if it can be combined with video surveillance in individuals who have sufficiently frequent attacks so that one of them is likely to occur during monitoring. Other techniques such as the use of special electrodes may be needed, for example when the attacks arise from the medial temporal lobe, which may produce little disturbance in the normal scalp electrodes.

The possibility of continuous minor epilepsy as the explanation for a confusional state or apparent dementia makes an EEG recording in search of 'sub-clinical' seizure activity appropriate in such circumstances. A particularly disorganized high voltage record (hypsarrythmia) supports the diagnosis of infantile spasms in children with brief salaam attacks coming in runs.

Recordings during seizures are rare but characteristic. In absence seizures there is symmetrical frontal 3 Hz spike and wave. Tonic fits are accompanied by generalized 10 Hz or faster activity. Tonic clonic seizures begin with 10 Hz activity which is then followed by slow activity or mixed slow waves and spikes.

The management of status epilepticus can be facilitated by the availability of EEG recording in the ITU. Once the patient has been sedated, paralyzed and ventilated, the only guide to whether seizure activity is still occurring is the EEG.

Antiepileptic drugs in therapeutic doses have little effect on the EEG, and it is not advisable to stop them in the mistaken belief that they artefactually normalize records. Overdosage is revealed by slowing of the record and this can be diagnostically useful. The EEG does not reliably predict the chance of safely stopping medication, except sometimes in children.

Dementia

EEG recordings can be of help in the assessment of dementia, both in excluding sub-clinical epilepsy and highlighting the possibility of a pseudodementia when the record is entirely normal. The record can be normal in the earliest stages of Alzheimer's disease, though reduction in alpha frequency and amplitude is usual. The likelihood of Creutzfeld–Jakob disease as a cause of rapidly progressive dementia is increased if the EEG develops repetitive stereotyped complexes (Figure 3.16). Weekly records may have to be planned as the characteristic changes are only seen at a certain stage in the evolution of the disease. It has been suggested that the diagnosis is unlikely if these changes do not emerge over a period of 10 weeks. Repetitive complexes appear to be typical of infections as they are also seen with herpes simplex virus encephalitis (Figure 3.17) and subacute sclerosing panencephalitis due to persistence of the measles virus. Their timing and distribution differs in these diverse conditions. Focal abnormalities in a demented patient can be seen when tumours, multiple infarcts or hydrocephalus are present.

Metabolic encephalopathy

Monitoring the functional changes in brain function in metabolic disorders that cause no structural (and hence imaging) abnormalities

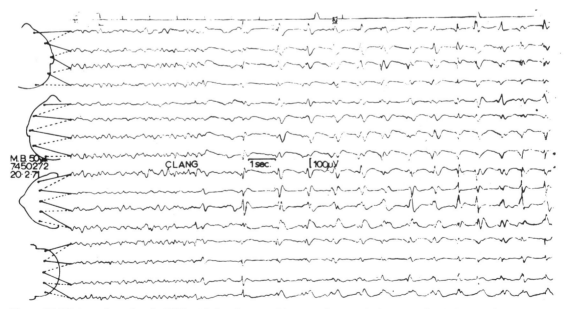

Figure 3.16 Sixteen-channel scalp EEG read showing repetitive complexes replacing normal activity in a dementing patient with Creutzfeld–Jakob disease.

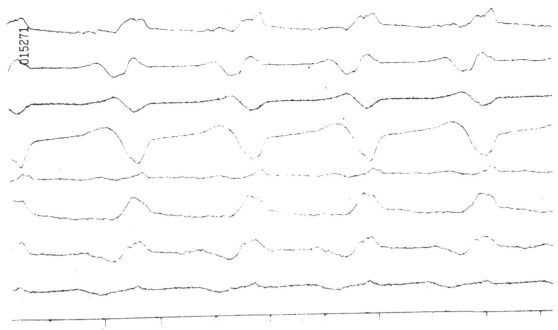

Figure 3.17 Eight channels from a scalp EEG record showing repetitive complexes from both right (top four channels) and left (lower four channels) temporal lobes with loss of all normal activity. Severe case of herpes simplex encephalitis. Calibration in seconds (lowest trace).

is another role for the EEG. Some causes of drowsiness and confusion, such as hepatic encephalopathy and renal failure, may produce triphasic waves in the EEG, such that the aetiology can be inferred from the tracings (Figure 3.18). In other situations the severity of metabolic brain derangement can be followed along with the response to treatment. Slowing of the alpha frequency, loss of its responsiveness to stimuli, and subsequent slowing to theta or delta frequencies parallels the severity of the metabolic derangement. The effect of protein restriction on the severity of hepatic encephalopathy, and the response of the EEG to manipulation of serum calcium levels are cases in point. Quantitative EEG indices of uraemic encephalopathy have been used to monitor the adequacy of dialysis protocols. In the operating theatre, EEG monitoring is used to document the level of anaesthesia and to detect ischaemic problems during procedures like carotid endarterectomy and coronary artery bypass surgery.

Cerebrovascular disease

Routine MRI and CT cannot always detect areas of ischaemic damage, and the distinction between deep lacunar infarction and embolic cortical infarction may figure in the choice of treatment. The EEG tends to be normal with small deep infarcts, but abnormal over a cortical lesion. Multiple foci of EEG abnormality in a demented individual raises the possibility of multi-infarct rather than Alzheimer's dementia.

Coma

The EEG can help in the assessment of comatose patients. Subclinical status epilepticus is readily identified, and repetitive complexes over one or both temporal lobes suggests herpes simplex encephalitis. If imaging has

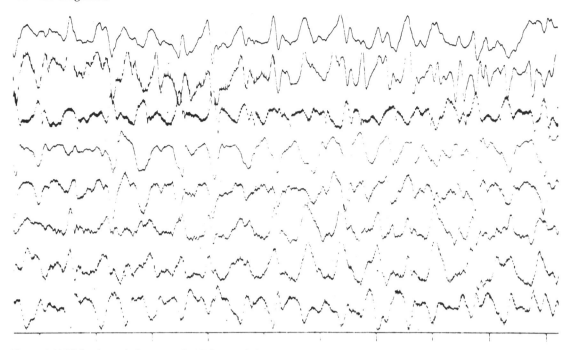

Figure 3.18 Eight channels from a scalp EEG record showing diffuse slow waves some of which are of triphasic pattern in a case of hepatic encephalopathy. Calibration in seconds (lowest trace).

not yet been carried out a focal abnormality in a comatose patient suggests (as it does in the alert subject) a mass lesion (Figure 3.19). A responsive record alerts the physician to the possibility of a locked-in state. The prognosis of coma due to hypoxic–ischaemic damage after cardiorespiratory arrest can be judged from the EEG. In the absence of drug effect and hypothermia a straight line EEG devoid of waveforms implies a hopeless outlook. A flat EEG is defined by the absence of any waveform above 2 μV when recorded by electrode pairs at least 10 cm apart with electrode impedances less than 10 000 ohms. Little chance of recovery exists if the EEG pattern is of alternating bursts of activity and moments of electrocerebral silence ('burst-suppression') (Figure 3.20). By contrast, any retention of responsive alpha rhythm implies a good prognosis. In brain death there is electrocerebral silence: a confirmatory rather than essential test.

Sleep disorders

EEG recordings are usually combined with monitoring of respiratory and eye movements to detect sleep apnoea as a cause of daytime sleepiness. The patient who snores excessively wakes frequently during the night as his airway collapses and obstructs. The EEG shows the arousal each time respiration is impeded. Positive pressure in a face mask is a highly successful treatment.

In narcolepsy associated with the HLA type DR2 patients fall asleep abruptly at inappropriate moments, for example during a meal, when their head falls into the soup, or during an interview for a job. EEGs show sleep onset with rapid eye movement sleep, a stage not normally entered in the first 90 minutes of normal sleep. These useful diagnostic features can be elicited by the expedient of repeatedly allowing the patient to fall

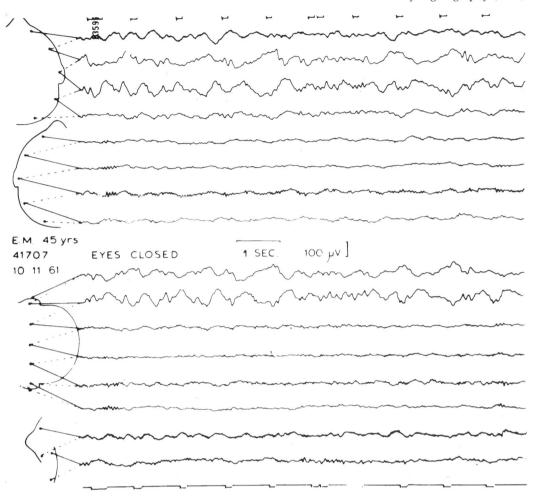

E.M. 45 yrs
41707   EYES CLOSED   1 SEC.   100 µV]
10 11 61

Figure 3.19 Sixteen-channel scalp EEG record showing focal slow wave abnormality over the right mid-temporal region due to a glioma.

asleep in a quiet environment (to measure sleep latency and to detect REM onset sleep). The same patients may describe cataplexy, in which a paroxysm of laughter precipitates a loss of muscle tone causing collapse or immobility.

Excessive daytime sleepiness in other patients proves to show no signs of apnoea or narcolepsy but may show short latency to sleep onset. Affective disorders, drug and alcohol all interfere with sleep patterns but polysomnographic recording is rarely required.

Electronystagmography (ENG)

Because of the existence of a standing potential between the front and back of the eyeball, electrodes on the skin around the orbits can be used to detect and record eye movements. This enables the effect of darkness and eye closure on nystagmus to be investigated. Horizontal nystagmus due to

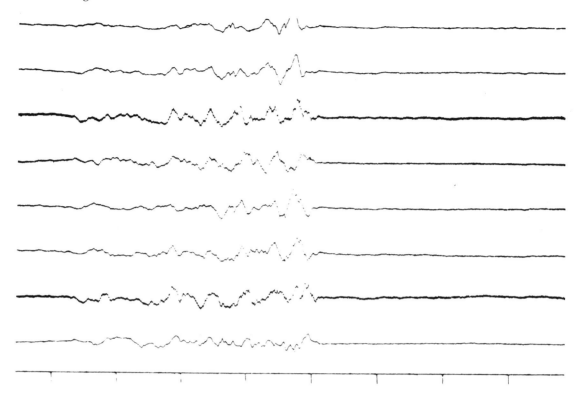

Figure 3.20 Eight channels from a scalp EEG record showing only intermittent evidence of cerebral activity — so called burst suppression pattern — of poor prognosis after hypoxic ischaemic damage. Calibration in seconds (lowest trace).

peripheral labyrinthine disease is enhanced in darkness; central brain-stem nystagmus is not. The rebound nystagmus of cerebellar disease as the eyes return to central fixation after an excursion is difficult to see at the bedside but clear on ENG recordings. Subclinical nystagmus can be detected in multiple sclerosis, for example.

Cerebrospinal fluid

Examination of the CSF is indicated in a few situations. Doing a good lumbar puncture is a skill worth acquiring for both the doctor's and patient's sake. The first move is to explain to the patient what is entailed, and to gain their consent. Stress that it is expected to be painless, as local anaesthetic will be used. Explain that the patient will be asked to stay in bed for a short while to allow the missing fluid to be replaced. If headache is discussed make sure that it is put in context. Whatever the patient has heard to the contrary, headache is by no means the rule (about 30%), and is usually simply dealt with by a day in bed with simple analgesics. It is due to a continuing loss of fluid through the puncture site in the dura. More serious complications like sixth nerve palsy, or an intracranial bleed or infection are very rare indeed.

The positioning of the patient is crucial to the ease of the procedure. The patient should lie on his side: for the right-handed doctor this will usually be the patient's left side. The patient should lie on the edge of the mattress where it is supported by the side frame of the bed. This prevents lateral sagging of the spine. The position for the patient to adopt is the foetal one with knees and legs bunched up under the chin. This opens the interspinous spaces, as seen from the back. The head does not have to be forced into a flexed posture. To keep the back vertical pillows should be placed between the knees. Next, the L3/4 space is felt by noting the level of the superior iliac spines, and by palpation. The area of the lumbar spine around this point is then sterilized and draped and the operator dons sterile gloves. A small bleb of local anaesthetic is injected into the skin at the point where the space between the vertebral spines can be felt. When this has begun to act infiltrate deeper with more anaesthetic. Whilst this is working it is wise to check that the LP 'set' is complete, that the manometer fits, etc. It is not a good moment to discover the lack of a tap or suitable sample bottles when the needle is already in place.

The disposable needle is then inserted. Usually a 20 gauge needle is chosen. Smaller needles are less likely to cause post-LP headache, but can be more difficult to insert and cannot be used if pressure measurements are crucial, as in cases of benign intracranial hypertension. Larger bore needles may be helpful in patients in whom it is known the procedure is technically difficult, as the reduced flexibility of the needle can make its manipulation easier. The needle is inserted with its bevel in the plane of the spine and its shaft strictly horizontal and angled slightly towards the patient's head. Some 'aim' for the umbilicus. If bone is struck, the needle is withdrawn to the subcutaneous region and re-angled before a new attempt is made. If the patient gets pain down the leg the needle is not quite in the midline and is irritating a nerve root. The needle is advanced slowly, held between thumb and index of the dominant hand.

When the path is correct the passage through the paraspinal ligament is felt, and there is a second give as the dura is broached. The stylet can then be withdrawn, when fluid should drip out spontaneously. If no fluid appears and the operator feels the needle is 'in', it is permissable to rotate the unprotected tip of the needle, but not to advance it unless

the stylet is in place, and not to attach a syringe and attempt to aspirate fluid. If neat blood appears due to a puncture of the venous plexus, the next space (L2/3 or 4/5) must be punctured. The venous plexus lies anteriorly so this mishap usually means the needle has been advanced too far. This is avoided by patiently checking by removing the stylet every 2 mm after crossing the ligament on the way in.

If no fluid is obtained (a dry tap), the procedure should be repeated in the sitting position with the patient leaning forward with their head on their folded arms on a support such as a bed table. If this too fails or great difficulty is encountered in finding the intervertebral space, perhaps in a fat patient, the possibility of carrying out the procedure under fluoroscopic control in the X-ray department should be discussed. If this too fails or is deemed impossible, for example in a patient with a fused lumbar spine, or is contraindicated in a patient with a suspected lumbar epidural abscess, CSF may be obtained by an expert using a lateral puncture at C1/2. Rarely the pressure is too low for fluid to escape spontaneously at lumbar puncture due to a total spinal block, for example by a spinal tumour or abscess. Such a patient will be paraplegic and will need neuroimaging and not an LP.

If the pressure is to be measured, attach the manometer. Ensure there is a free communication by observing movement of the meniscus with respiration and record the height of the CSF column. The pressure is normally under 200 mm of CSF. If the pressure is higher than this, it is important to check that this is not artefactual due to the patient being in a tense state and perhaps doing a Valsalva manoeuvre. Get the patient to straighten his legs slowly to reduce abdominal pressure and see if the pressure is still high. Do not conclude a pressure of 200–250 mm of CSF is abnormal until 5 minutes have elapsed and the patient has been made comfortable and as calm as possible. Some 5% of the normal population can have a pressure in this range, even then. Pressure readings are unreliable in the sitting position.

The contents of the manometer are run into collecting specimen bottles. A few millilitres are run into each of three bottles, and a fluoride bottle is used to acquire a sample for CSF sugar estimation. A blood sugar must also be taken at this time or the CSF level cannot be interpreted. The CSF level is normally not less than 40% of the blood level. If fungal cultures are to be done then larger volumes of fluid will be needed. The puncture site is pressed on briefly and a plaster put on the skin — as long as the patient is not allergic to it!

Lumbar punctures should not be done if there is local sepsis near the puncture site, if the patient has a coagulopathy or is thrombocytopenic. Plasma or platelet transfusion is necessary if the puncture is vital in these circumstances. If they are on heparin it should be stopped for 6 hours, and not restarted for another 4.

The routine assay of CSF protein and cell content requires prompt handling. The identification of cell type, including malignant cells requires inspection of the fresh fluid. Only urgent specimens (e.g. in meningitis and sub-arachnoid haemorrhage) should be taken out of hours. If the fluid is blood stained the sample should be centrifuged immediately and the supernatant inspected for discoloration and preferably subjected to spectroscopy (to identify the presence of bilirubin). The normal fluid is water or 'gin' clear. An increase in protein or white cells can make it cloudy. The protein is increased with breakdown of the blood–brain barrier due to inflammation, trauma, or tumours, though rarely a metabolic condition is responsible (diabetes, hypothyroidism, renal failure, hypercalcaemia). Polymorphs appear with acute infections, lymphocytes with chronic infections and

those due to viruses, and eosinophils with rare parasitic infection. A low CSF sugar is seen with bacterial, fungal, and carcinomatous meningitis. It is also seen in neurosyphilis and sarcoidosis. Antibody titres are diagnostic in cryptococcal, Borrelia, and syphilitic infections.

Meningitis/encephalitis

The diagnosis of meningitis or encephalitis requires the demonstration of a pleocytosis in the fluid and the microbiological diagnosis of the specific cause of such infections is also dependent on staining and culture of the fluid. Patients with febrile headache, photophobia and meningism (meningitis suspected), perhaps with confusion, disorientation, epilepsy or focal deficit (encephalitis suspected) should therefore be lumbar punctured, preferably after brain scanning, to eliminate rival diagnoses such as a brain abscess when a LP would be hazardous. If scanning is not immediately available, and especially if the patient has papilloedema, focal signs, or depressed consciousness, blood cultures should be obtained and antibiotics started without a lumbar puncture.

The differential diagnosis of bacterial, tuberculous, fungal, viral and malignant meningitis is suggested by the absolute and differential white cell count, protein level and sugar content. CSF lactate levels over 3.5 mmolar are also suggestive of bacterial meningitis. PCR for viruses and perhaps TB and the search for cryptococcal antigens can make the

Table 3.1 Differential diagnosis of meningitis from the CSF

	POLYS	LYMPHS	PROT	GLUC	MICROB	OTHER
BACT	+++	+	+	− ↓	+	Lactate +
VIRAL	+/−	++	+	−	+	PCR
TB	+/−	++	+	− ↓	+	PCR ?
FUNGI	+/−	++	+	− ↓	+	Antigen (cryptococcal)
MALIG	−	+/−	+	− − ↓↓	−	Cytology

+ = Increased
↓ = Reduced
− = Normal
Microb = Microbiological stains/cultures
PCR = Polymerase chain reaction

microbiological diagnosis when simple inspection of stained samples is unsuccessful. If the sample is contaminated by traumatic blood at the time of puncture, the counts can be corrected by subtracting one white cell for every 700–1000 red cells. The CSF protein can be similarly compensated for contamination by subtracting 1 mg protein/dl for every 700 red cells. The IgG/protein ratio rises 0.037 for every 3333 red cells.

If malignant meningitis is suspected, more than one lumbar puncture may be needed. The chance of finding carcinomatous or lymphomatous cells in the fluid are about 25–50% on the first occasion rising to 75% by the time three punctures have been done. Fresh 'warm' samples give the cytologist the best chance of a positive identification.

Subarachnoid haemorrhage

If CT scanning fails to reveal subarachnoid blood in a patient with severe headache of sudden onset (with or without meningism and photophobia), lumbar puncture is indicated so that a spectroscopic analysis can look for the presence of haemoglobin breakdown products in the fluid. The distinction between a blood stained CSF and one contaminated by trauma due to the needle depends on the progressive decline in red cells in successive bottles collected, the presence of discoloration of the supernatant after centrifugation (xanthochromia), and on the spectroscopy. If the LP is carried out too soon (a few hours) after the onset of a subarachnoid haemorrhage blood and its products may not have reached the lumbar fluid. If the clinical event is some 3 weeks in the past, it will usually be too late for even spectroscopic evidence of a bleed.

Multiple sclerosis

Oligoclonal IgG is detected in the CSF of 95% of patients with multiple sclerosis. This is still a useful guide to the diagnosis, for example in a patient with optic neuritis or myelitis. MRI in such patients may reveal many cerebral white matter lesions but is not always conclusive and may not be available. The differential diagnosis of the presence of oligoclonal bands includes sarcoidosis, neurosyphilis, lupus, HIV infection, herpes encephalitis, some cases of carcinomatous cerebellar degeneration, and by contamination by an abnormal plasma protein. A paired blood sample should therefore always accompany the CSF specimen when oligoclonal bands are being sought.

Guillain–Barré syndrome

Acute inflammatory demyelinating neuropathy shows a diagnostically confirmatory elevated protein without pleocytosis in patients with a short history of peripheral parasthesiae and limb weakness, with or without facial and respiratory weakness. The fluid may be normal in the first week. Oligoclonal bands or a pleocytosis suggest the patient may have underlying HIV infection.

Neurosyphilis

Patients with positive syphilis serology need examination of the CSF for evidence of active neurosyphilis with pleocytosis and positive serology in the fluid. More than five white cells, a protein over 0.4, and positive FTA indicates neurological involvement and the need for treatment. Patients with epilepsy or dementia, or young cases of stroke may fall into this group.

Neuroimaging

The roles of CT and MRI are complementary, and their usefulness will be discussed in the main areas in which evidence is sought for structural brain or spinal disease.

Head injury

CT scanning is the first imaging procedure of choice because it is so sensitive in the acute stages to the presence of blood, and because scanning is rapid which means it is more likely to produce images of diagnostic quality in a restless patient. If necessary, it is possible to scan paralysed and ventilated patients.

Contusion is seen as ill-defined low density in the cortico-subcortical region due to focal oedema. If the contusion is haemorrhagic then the abnormal area is of high density. Such areas are often in the frontobasal region or at the tip of the temporal lobe. The main importance of imaging patients with head injury is to detect haematomas that are potentially damaging due to mass effect and which need evacuating.

Extradural haematomas are biconvex areas of high density over the cerebral surface. They often overlie the area of fracture especially when that affects the middle meningeal artery. By contrast, the subdural haematoma is a concave convex area. It too is hyperdense in the first three weeks or so. Chronic subdural haematomas (which may present up to 9 months after the injury) become of low density after those first weeks (Figure 3.21). Intracerebral haematomas are hyperdense areas within brain substance and are only seen in major head injury (Figure 3.22). Subarachnoid blood is common with increased density in cisterns, between the hemispheres, and over the convexity.

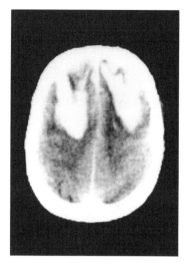

Figure 3.22 CT scan in head-injured patient showing bilateral frontal haematomas.

Although MRI is very sensitive to contusion, it is less sensitive to the presence of blood in the first 24 hours.

Strokes

The differential diagnosis of cerebral haemorrhage from infarction is most easily decided in the first days after stroke by CT scanning (Figures 3.23 and 3.24). MRI is more sensitive to areas of infarction which may be missed by early CT (Figure 3.25). MRI particularly has the 'edge' in the posterior fossa in the detec-

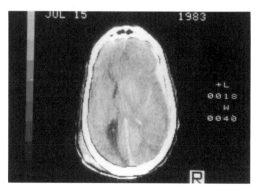

Figure 3.21 CT scan. A subdural haematoma is causing shift of the midline to the left.

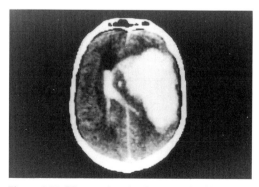

Figure 3.23 CT scan showing large cerebral haematoma. Blood has entered the ventricular system.

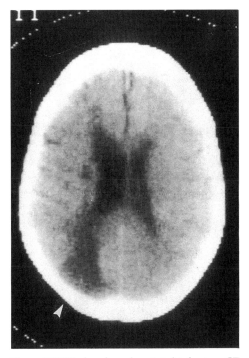

Figure 3.24 Wedge shaped occipital infarct on CT scan on left.

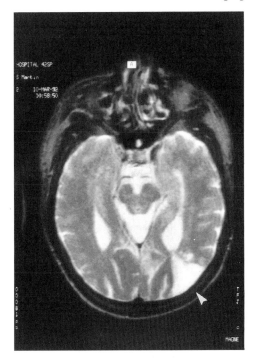

Figure 3.25 Similar infarct on T2 weighted MRI on right. Note second infarct alongside lateral ventricle which is of lacunar size.

tion of infarcts, and in documenting lacunar infarction or more diffuse white matter changes associated with small vessel disease.

Parenchymatous haemorrhage is a circumscribed area of high density on CT with mass effect and in some cases ventricular haemorrhage is associated with it. Pontine or cerebellar haemorrhage may cause hydrocephalus by blocking the aqueduct. By contrast, infarcts are often wedge-shaped areas of low signal with the base of the cone at the cortex, and within a vascular territory. After about 3 weeks haemorrhages are also of low density. At this stage MRI can identify the presence of blood products and is better at making the distinction. MRI is also better at 'seeing' vessels in lesions like AVMs thanks to a signal 'void' due to flowing blood.

Haemorrhagic infarction shows patchy high density within the low density area on CT scans, as often seen with cardiogenic infarcts. MRI shows mixed signal densities in this context and is more sensitive to small amounts of blood products.

Tumours

Meningiomas on CT are enhancing areas of high density of circumscribed outline in characteristic sites (interhemispheric, subfrontal, sphenoidal ridge). On MRI they are often isodense but enhance (Figure 3.26). CT is perhaps preferred in their detection, but MRI gives the surgeon additional information about their blood supply.

Gliomas appear on CT (Figure 3.27) as areas of low density with mass effect and enhancement due to a damaged blood–brain barrier in the more aggressive tumours. Such enhancement is usually irregular and quite unlike the homogenous blush of the meningioma. Oligodendrogliomas are usually calcified on CT, and metastases which are often multiple usually have intense enhancement and associated oedema (Figure 3.28).

MRI (Figure 3.29) is better able to see tumours in the posterior fossa, including

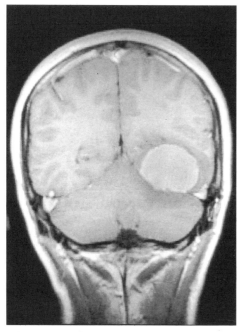

Figure 3.26 MRI T1 weighted after gadolinium enhancement showing a large meningioma — see also Figure 3.39.

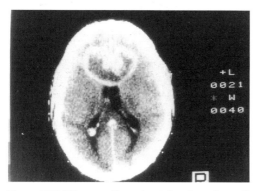

Figure 3.27 CT scan with contrast showing a butterfly shaped enhancing glioma in the frontal lobes. The patient presented with dementia.

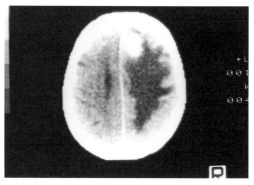

Figure 3.28 A small frontal metastasis with extensive hemispheric oedema on CT.

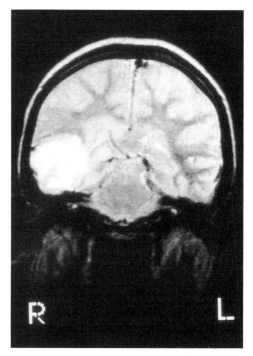

Figure 3.29 MRI coronal T2 weighted image with a temporal lobe glioma.

small acoustic neuromas (Figure 3.30) which are best detected by MRI with gadolinium enhancement. Gadolinium may show up granulomas such as those due to sarcoidosis (Figure 3.31). Pituitary microadenomas are well seen by MRI as small areas of low signal on T1 images. Macroadenomas are well demonstrated by MRI (Figure 3.32) and particularly when there is destruction of the pituitary fossa by enhanced CT.

Abscesses

These are well seen by CT when fully developed with ring enhancement due to the

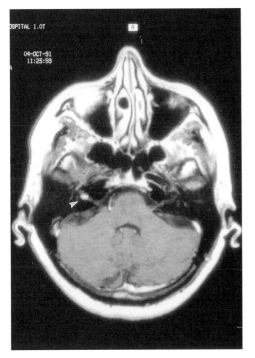

Figure 3.30 MRI T1 weighted after gadolinium injection showing a bright enhancing neuroma on the acoustic nerve on the left (arrowed).

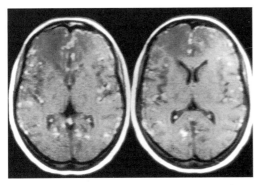

Figure 3.31 MRI T1 weighted after gadolinium showing multiple enhancing granulomas (sarcoidosis).

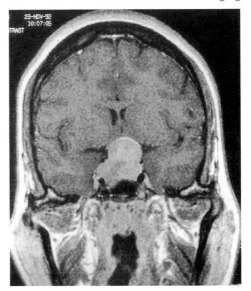

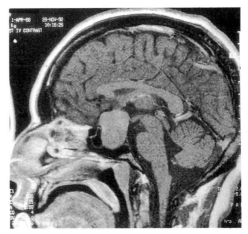

Figure 3.32 MRI T1 after gadolinium showing large pituitary tumour that has spread into the cavernous sinus and into the suprasellar region.

abscess wall. MRI is more sensitive to the inflammatory oedema so detects areas of cerebritis more readily (Figure 3.33a). Patients with multiple abscesses may have only one lesion on CT, but several on MRI. The differential diagnosis includes multiple metastases, and tuberculosis, and can be very difficult. Both techniques reveal extracerebral collections of pus (Figure 3.33b).

Encephalitis

By choice one would chose MRI to identify inflammatory oedema, for example in the temporal lobes of a case of herpes simplex encephalitis (HSE) with areas of high signal on T2 (Figure 3.34). CT shows low density in the same cases, but less reliably. Such changes in a case of encephalitis point strongly to HSE

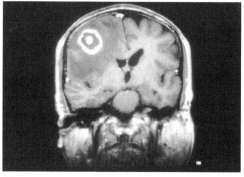

(a)

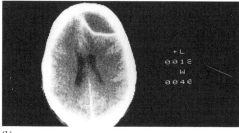

(b)

Figure 3.33 (a) T1 MRI after gadolinium showing ring enhancing abscess with surrounding oedema. (b) CT scan showing extradural collection of pus in a patient with frontal sinusitis.

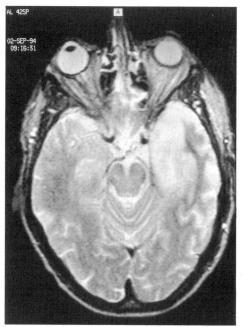

Figure 3.34 MRI T2 weighted showing inflammatory oedema of temporal lobe due to herpes simplex encephalitis.

even before other diagnostic methods are available.

Dementia

The rationale for the investigation of demented patients even when they have no clinical signs of focal brain disease is to detect treatable causes such as hydrocephalus (Figure 3.35), and tumours (Figure 3.28). Most however will have only atrophy on CT or MRI with enlarged ventricles more reliable than sulcal dilatation (Figure 3.36). Others will have multiple infarcts and/or white matter changes believed to be ischaemic in aetiology. Caudate atrophy can be striking in Huntington's disease (basal ganglia changes are also seen in Wilson's disease, prompting copper studies if these have not already been made in response to the onset of a movement

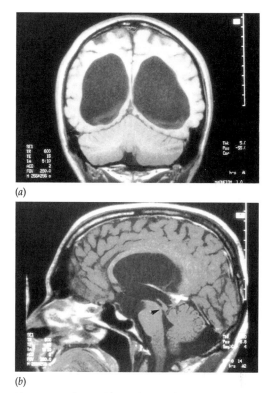

(a)

(b)

Figure 3.35 Coronal MRI showing (a) grossly dilated ventricles in a patient with aqueduct stenosis; (b) arrowed.

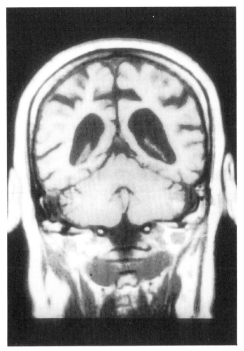

Figure 3.36 MRI showing dilated ventricles and sulci in demented subject.

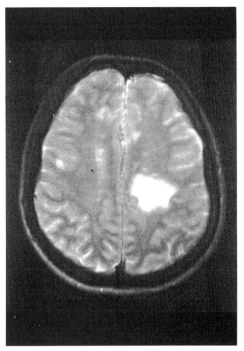

Figure 3.37 MRI T2 weighted in case of multiple sclerosis. A large plaque is seen on the right.

Multiple sclerosis

CT rarely detects large areas of demyelination. MRI has revolutionized the diagnosis of MS as, though not specific, it is highly sensitive to the presence of plaques. They appear as areas of high signal on T2 around the borders of ventricles and in the corpus callosum (Figure 3.37). On sagittal images they appear linear and orientated like sunrays from the callosal margin towards the cortex. Active lesions, whether clinically overt or not, enhance with gadolinium.

Cerebral aneurysms

MR angiography is sensitive enough to screen asymptomatic patients for aneurysms, for example when there is a family history of sub-arachnoid haemorrhage or polycystic kidneys with which they are associated. When the patient has had a proven bleed (Figure 3.38), arterial angiography is required with injections of contrast material in all four vessels. When such films detect more than one aneurysm, radiological clues as to which one has bled are available from the site of blood on

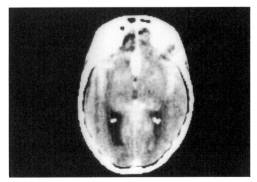

Figure 3.38 CT scan showing subarachnoid blood after subarachnoid haemorrhage.

the CT scan and the presence of spasm of vessels around the bleeding site.

High density lesions on CT

These are generally due to blood or calcification. Calcification in the falx, the choroid plexus, the pineal and basal ganglia can be normal, but is also seen in tumours (oligodendrogliomas, craniopharyngiomas, and some meningiomas), and AVMs. It is also encountered in tuberculous and CMV infections, and in the scars of old sites of trauma.

Low density lesions on CT

Infarcts, tumours, abscesses, old haematomas, arachnoid cysts and lipomas all appear of low density. The differential diagnosis depends on site, shape, and pattern of enhancement, e.g. gyral in cortical infarction, irregular in tumours (Figure 3.28), ring in abscesses (Figure 3.33).

Spine

MRI is the procedure of choice to investigate spinal cord diseases including spondylosis, disc prolapse, tumours (Figure 3.39 a,b) and myelitis. Congenital abnormalities at the foramen magnum such as cerebellar ectopia with syringomyelia, or spinal dysraphism in the lumbar region are well demonstrated. Myelography, with its need for lumbar puncture, and risk of deterioration in the case of cord compression (Fib 3.39 b) is still appropriate when MRI is unavailable, the patient is unable to tolerate the magnet, or movement degrades the images too much for diagnosis. Compression of the cord can be distinguished from an intrinsic spinal cord tumour by the swelling of the tumour-bearing cord. An intradural mass such as a neurofibroma displaces the cord (Figure 3.40). Extradural masses may just obliterate the canal with little lateral

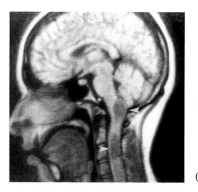

(a)

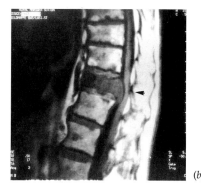

(b)

Figure 3.39 (a) Extensive glioma of the spinal cord revealed by T1 MRI in sagittal plane (arrowed). (b) Compression of cord by vertebral metastasis (arrowed).

deviation of the cord. If contrast material is injected, CT slices are obtained as well as routine films during screening. Plain CT also has a role in malignant disease as it is sensitive to the presence of vertebral disease.

CT or MRI?

CT is preferred to MRI for acute cerebral haemorrhage, subarachnoid haemorrhage, acute head injury, calcified tumours and bone disease. MRI is preferred to CT in cerebral ischaemia, multiple sclerosis, arteriovenous malformations, posterior fossa problems, white matter disease, and spinal cord disease.

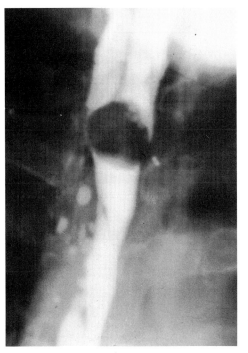

Figure 3.40 Spinal cord tumour (neurofibroma) revealed by contrast myelography.

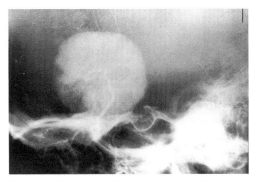

Figure 3.41 The external carotid artery has been injected, revealing the vascular blush of a frontal meningioma.

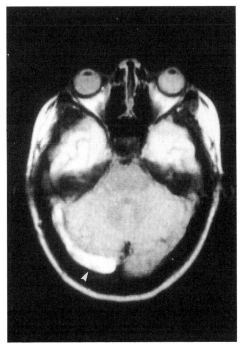

Figure 3.42 MRI T1 showing high signal from thrombosed sigmoid and lateral sinuses in case of venous thrombosis (arrowed).

X-ray angiography

Opacification of cerebral vessels by intra-arterial injections of radiopaque iodine compounds is rarely needed in the identification of brain tumours thanks to the sensitivity of CT and MR scanning (Figure 3.41). It is still pertinent in the investigation of angiomas and cerebral venous thrombosis though MR and MR angiography is also usurping this role to some extent (Figure 3.42). The need for four vessel angiography to search for aneurysms in a case of subarachnoid haemorrhage has already been mentioned (Figure 3.43).

Angiography is still the gold standard investigation in the search for operable carotid artery stenosis in cases of TIA and recovering stroke (Figure 3.44). Screening is by ultrasound, MR angiography, or intravenous angiography. Concordance of two non-invasive tests makes for a reliable estimate of disease, but MRA alone or Duplex imaging alone may give a false estimate of the extent of arterial wall disease.

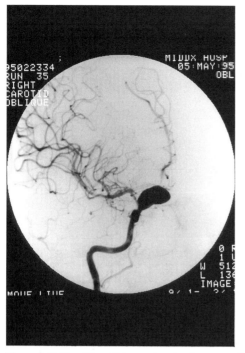

Figure 3.43 Carotid angiogram showing large carotid aneurysm which had produced visual loss due to chiasmal compression.

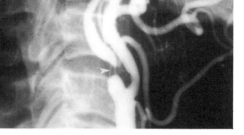

Figure 3.44 Angiogram showing stenosis of the origin of the internal carotid artery in a patient with TIAs.

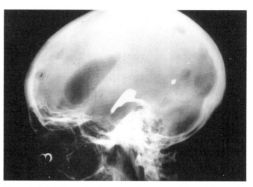

Figure 3.45 Ventriculogram showing dilated lateral ventricles filled partially with air above and a dilated 3rd ventricle due to an obstructed aqueduct outlined by myodil below.

Air and myodil ventriculography

These techniques are now only of historical interest. They depended on the injection into the lateral ventricle via a burr hole of air which floated above the CSF, and/or oily myodil which sunk below it (Figure 3.45). Tumours and obstructions in CSF pathways were thereby demonstrated. In air encephalography air was injected via a lumbar puncture and allowed to outline CSF containing spaces in the head. As well as outlining deep tumours it was used to distinguish between atrophy (dilated ventricles and sulci) and hydrocephalus (isolated dilatation of the ventricles). These roles have all been taken over by CT and MR scanning.

Investigation of bladder dysfunction

MRI scanning of the lumbosacral cord has become the investigation of choice if a lesion at this level is suspected. Neurophysiological investigations have proved to be of value in recognizing the changes of chronic reinnervation that occur in either the urethral or anal sphincter as an early feature of multiple system atrophy. Urethral sphincter EMG is currently the only means of demonstrating an abnormality in young women with urinary retention without any general neurological features.

Cystometry, the filling of the bladder and measurement of the intravesical and intrarectal pressure, is a valuable investigation for demonstrating the pathophysiological behaviour of the bladder. It must be emphasized, however, that it is not diagnostic in terms of the site of the neurological lesion. By far the commonest finding in patients with neurogenic incontinence is hyperreflexia, but the cystometric appearances can be similar with this, whatever the site of the lesion. Detrusor sphincter dyssinergia is technically difficult to demonstrate but its presence would reasonably be expected in any patient with a paraparesis.

In terms of management, recognizing incomplete emptying is important. Incomplete bladder emptying can be demonstrated using either urethral catheterization following voiding, or a simple ultrasound machine. The combination of an ultrasound measurement of post-micturition residual volume and measurement of urine flow rates together make a well tolerated set of investigations which, if normal, go some way towards excluding significant neurogenic bladder dysfunction.

Tissue biopsies

Muscle biopsy

This is often indicated in the pursuit of a diagnosis in patients with a myopathic distribution of weakness in whom there is no systemic disease or medication to explain it. Muscle biopsy may also be revealing in patients with CNS disease (vasculitis, mitochondrial diseases).

Polymyositis is detected by the combination of muscle fibre necrosis and inflammatory cellular infiltrate. Dystrophies also have muscle fibre degeneration, but there is also evidence of regeneration and proliferation of connective tissue elements.

Mitochondrial cytopathy which may present with encephalopathy, strokes or brain-

stem signs with or without muscle weakness, may show ragged red fibres due to the abnormal staining properties of fibres with abnormal mitochondria.

Type 2 fibre atrophy is common to many toxic or metabolic myopathies such as those related to steroids, or alcohol abuse.

Nerve biopsy

There is little to be gained by biopsy in axonal neuropathies, but the degree of demyelination and remyelination in those with chronic demyelinating neuropathies may be helpful. In addition, inflammatory cell infiltration, immune complex deposition and amyloid can also be detected. Hypertrophic changes are seen in hereditary neuropathies including Refsums, Charcot–Marie–Tooth, in chronic inflammatory demyelinating neuropathy, leprosy, amyloidosis, neurofibromatosis and acromegaly. Inflammatory cells are common to leprous neuropathy and sarcoidosis, for example. Sarcoidosis shows granulomas without necrosis as in other sites; leprosy the combination of epithelioid cells and giant cells. Some toxic neuropathies can be diagnosed by particular features such as axonal ballooning.

In the case of a mononeuritis multiplex, biopsy may reveal the causative vasculitis in the vasa nervorum.

Brain biopsy

This may be indicated in the case of mass lesions to establish the nature of tumour or abscess, and in cases of leukodystrophies when there are no abnormalities on metabolic screening. Meningeal biopsy has a role in the diagnosis of some vasculitides confined to the nervous system. Biopsy carries a risk of morbidity, including that due to haemorrhage, so it is now rare to consider it in degenerative conditions such as Alzheimer's disease.

Further reading

BINNIE, C.D. and PRIOR, P.F. (1994) Electroencephalography. *J. Neurol. Neurosurg. Psychiatry*, 57, 1308-1319.

BINNIE, C.D., COOPER, R., FOWLER, C.J., MAGUIERE, F. and PRYOR, P.F. (1995) *Clinical Neurophysiology. EMG, Nerve Conduction and Evoked Potentials*. Butterworth-Heinemann, Oxford.

HALLIDAY, M. (1993) *Evoked Potentials in Clinical Testing*. Churchill Livingstone, Edinburgh.

HUGHES, J.R. (1994) *EEG in Clinical Practice*. Butterworth-Heinemann, London.

PERKIN, G.D. (1988) *Diagnostic Tests in Neurology*. Chapman and Hall, London.

PROVENZALE, J.M. and TAVERAS, J.M. (1994) *Clinical Cases in Neuroradiology*. Lea and Fieberger, Philadelphia.

Index